Male Fertility Patterns and Determinants

THE SPRINGER SERIES ON

DEMOGRAPHIC METHODS AND POPULATION ANALYSIS

Series Editor

KENNETH C. LAND

Duke University

In recent decades, there has been a rapid development of demographic models and methods and an explosive growth in the range of applications of population analysis. This series seeks to provide a publication outlet both for high-quality textual and expository books on modern techniques of demographic analysis and for works that present exemplary applications of such techniques to various aspects of population analysis.

Topics appropriate for the series include:

- General demographic methods
- Techniques of standardization
- Life table models and methods
- Multistate and multiregional life tables, analyses and projections
- Demographic aspects of biostatistics and epidemiology
- Stable population theory and its extensions
- Methods of indirect estimation
- Stochastic population models
- Event history analysis, duration analysis, and hazard regression models
- Demographic projection methods and population forecasts
- Techniques of applied demographic analysis, regional and local population estimates and projections
- Methods of estimation and projection for business and health care applications
- Methods and estimates for unique populations such as schools and students

Volumes in the series are of interest to researchers, professionals, and students in demography, sociology, economics, statistics, geography and regional science, public health and health care management, epidemiology, biostatistics, actuarial science, business, and related fields.

For further volumes:
http://www.springer.com/series/6449

Li Zhang

Male Fertility Patterns and Determinants

Springer

Dr. Li Zhang
L. Douglas Wilder School of Government
and Public Affairs
Virginia Commonwealth University
923 West Franklin Street
Richmond, VA 23284-2028
USA
lzhang5@vcu.edu

ISSN 1389-6784
ISBN 978-90-481-8938-0 e-ISBN 978-90-481-8939-7
DOI 10.1007/978-90-481-8939-7
Springer Dordrecht Heidelberg London New York

Printed on acid-free paper

Springer is part of Springer Science+Business Media (www.springer.com)

I dedicate this book to my father,
Jianguo Zhang and to my mother,
Yanqing Shi.

Preface

The declining pattern of fertility has become universal in recent decades. Demographers and sociologists have explored such a pattern and have showed a variety of social and demographic factors that could have possibly caused fertility changes in various nations. As such, a number of fertility theories have been built to explain fertility variation. These studies and theories, however, have focused almost exclusively on the roles and patterns of females and their reproductive behaviors. Males have been largely ignored in sociological and demographic studies of fertility. Indeed, the majority of existing work on male fertility is primarily medical and biological in orientation.

Thus far, three books that have been published in sociology and demography on male fertility: Fertility and the Male Life-Cycle in the Era of Fertility Decline, edited by Caroline Bledsoe, Susan Lerner and Jane I. Guyer, Oxford University Press, 2000; Transitions to Adulthood in Europe, edited by Martine Corijn and Eric Klijzing, Kluwer Academic Publishers, 2001; and Dynamics of Human Reproduction by James W. Wood, Aldine De Gruyter Press, 1994. These books devote their attentions to the changing patterns of fatherhood and paternity in a variety of social contexts, the patterns and determinants of men and women as they enter into marital unions and start to have children in the European continent, and the natural and proximate determinants of men's fertility, respectively. These three books represent the pioneer research on male fertility and its related issues, which has considerably extended our understanding of men's status and roles in childbearing and family formation.

This current manuscript differentiates it from the above books in the following manners: First, this study expands the research scope on male fertility to the Eastern societies, such as Taiwan. The analysis provides a picture of the fertility patterns and determinants of males in a variety of social contexts, in contrast to other existing studies which are geographically limited. Second, the data used to conduct the analysis come from several newest available national databases. Third, the study goes beyond descriptive analysis to explore the multivariate relationship between male fertility and a number of factors. The gender differences in fertility shown in the books are also tested through statistical models. Fourth, this research combines cross-sectional and longitudinal analyses, aggregate and individual level analyses together to examine the subject matter, which directs possible pathways of future research.

The purpose of the book is to explore a broad range of factors that differentiate male fertility patterns and results from their female counterparts so that to challenge the female primacy assumption in fertility studies. In this manuscript, the book addresses such questions as: Do male and female fertility outcomes differ across nations and over time? Whether a variety of factors determine male and female fertility results in the same manner? What have caused the male and female fertility differentials? How do findings of this research benefit current family planning programs in both high and low fertility countries?

The book commences with a review of the existing literature on male fertility and the possible reasons that account for why men have been ignored in fertility studies. The study then presents an empirical analysis of male fertility by contrasting male and female fertility at both aggregate and individual levels. At the aggregate level, the book examines the changing pattern of male fertility rates as compared to female fertility rates in 43 countries and locations, particularly in Taiwan. The data used for aggregate level analysis come from the 2001 United Nations *Demographic Yearbook* and the 1964–2004 *Taiwan-Fukien Demographic Yearbooks* and the 2004 *National Statistics Reports* by the Statistics Bureau of Republic of China. The individual level analysis explores the fertility determinants of men as compared to those of women through analyzing data from the 2002 National Survey of Family Growth (NSFG) conducted in the United States. The book devotes particular attention to Taiwan and the United States due to their readily available male fertility data.

The results show that male and female fertility differ in rates and determinants in various social contexts, which clearly suggests that fertility variation cannot be entirely understood without given equal consideration to males. The book also proposes a number of reasons to explain male and female fertility differentials in rates. The book further illustrates the factors that differentiate male and female fertility outcomes. The implications drawn from this research suggest additional research attention be focused on the role and commitments of men when considering factors leading to decisions about bearing and rearing children.

Since this book studies male fertility and addresses men's role in family planning and fertility transition, the book will be of interest to a variety of readers. Scholars of fertility and family studies may find this research cutting-edge because this is one of the few frontier studies that examine men's childbearing. This book can also be used as a textbook in graduate and upper-division undergraduate sociology and demography core courses. Beyond the classroom, the book would also be of significant interest to a general audience, including policy makers who are interested in the topics of family planning, childbearing and rearing, gender and family issues, and population policy making.

Parts of the present volume have been adapted or excerpted from previously published work of the author. Chapter 5 is based on Li Zhang, Dudley L. Poston, Jr., and Chiung-Fang Chang. 2010. "Male and Female Fertility in Taiwan." In *The Family and Social Change in Chinese Societies*, edited by Dudley L. Poston, Jr., and Wenshan Yang, Rachel Traut Cortes, Heather Terrell Kincannon, and Cathy

Ruey-Ling Chu. New York: Springer Publisher, forthcoming. Chapter 7 is based on Li Zhang, 2008. "Religious Affiliation, Religiosity, and Male and Female Fertility." *Demographic Research*, Vol. 18: 233–262, used here with permission of *Demographic Research*.

Richmond, VA Li Zhang

Acknowledgments

This book represents several years of my research on male fertility while I was working on my Ph.D. at Texas A&M University (TAMU) and while I am serving an Assistant Professor at Virginia Commonwealth University (VCU) and a visiting research fellow at National University of Singapore. When I researched and wrote this book, a variety of people have offered their insights, assistance, support and encouragement. In acknowledging their contributions, it is perhaps appropriate to start at the beginning. In this regard, special thanks are owed first to Professor Dudley L. Poston, Jr. who has been both my mentor and friend at TAMU. He led me to the field of demography and provided me valuable guidance and tremendous help when I worked on this male fertility research. The book would not have been possible without his guidance and support. Dr. Mark Fossett, Dr. Alex McIntosh, Dr. Rogelio Saenz, and Dr. Don Albrecht spent their precious time on reading and commenting various chapters and drafts of this book. Dr. Lu Zheng and Dr. Jeff Ackerman also provided valuable advice on the methodology part of this book. I appreciate their enormous support to this manuscript.

A very special note of thanks also goes to several of my colleagues at VCU. Dr. John Mahoney, Dr. Jimmy Chen, Dr. Weiping Wu, Dr. Jennifer Johnson, Dr. Julie Honnold all offered their support, insights and suggestions. Particularly, I want to thank Dr. Nelson Wikstrom and Dr. Diana Scully who suggested important changes through reading the book prospectus and several chapters of the book. Dr. Nelson Wikstrom and Dr. Mike Leiber read through the manuscript and suggested valuable refinements and editorial changes, which ultimately contributed to a more cohesive and organized book. Dr. Sarah Jane Brubaker read and commented the "cohabitation and male fertility" chapter, which raised new issues and challenged some assumptions and conclusions of the chapter. Her effort ultimately contributed to a more solid book chapter.

My heartfelt thanks also go to my family, especially my parents, for their understanding and love throughout my time working on this manuscript. My gratitude is also extended to my friends Tuan Doan, Hai Zhao, Guiqing Liu, Zhixuan Zhao, Huitao Yang, and Nadia Flores. This book is as much theirs as it is mine.

I want to express my deepest appreciation to Elisabeth Groninger and Tony Love for proofreading my book chapters. Their comments and efforts are greatly appreciated. Thanks also go to Evelien Bakker and Bernadette Deelen at Springer, who have helped me along the way, have always been available to discuss emerging issues and questions, and have been a great pleasure to work with. I also appreciate the anonymous reviewers. Their comments have been extremely helpful to refine this manuscript.

Contents

List of Figures

List of Tables

Part I
Introduction

Chapter 1
Introduction and Overview

The twentieth century was witness to dramatic fertility changes, both in the industrial north and the less developed south. In the industrial north, fertility declined to below replacement levels in many countries during the Great Depression; it then rose due to the postwar "baby boom." Fertility in the south has been remained higher than that in the north. Coupled with declining death rates, high fertility rates in the south led to a population explosion during the 1950s and 1960s. As the century came to an end, fertility decline was shown almost everywhere and population growth was no longer a major concern. Instead, the below replacement level fertility has given rise to fears of depopulation in some European and Asian countries with lowest-low fertility rates. Significant social changes occurred as consequences of fertility decline. These changes include the declines in "the size of families, sibships and households, the number of close relatives, and the years spent as parents of small children" (Morgan & Hagewen, 2005, p. 230). In the process of fertility decline and the subsequent social changes, men's role and participation nevertheless, have hardly been considered by most demographic literature.

Fertility theories that are used to explain changes in human fertility have rarely included men. Prominent explanations of fertility change include the proximate determinants theory (Bongaarts, 1994), demographic transition theory (Notestein, 1953), wealth flows theory (Caldwell, 1982), human ecological theory (Poston & Frisbie, 2005), political economic theory (Greenhalgh, 1990) and diffusion theory (Watkins, 1991), are almost exclusively geared toward women and their roles in the process of childbearing. Men are seldom included in the existing fertility theories.

In addition to fertility theories, empirical analyses of fertility also show a strong female-dominated tradition. When I used POPLINE, a digital achieve of literature on reproductive health, to conduct a review of the literature on the topic of fertility, the search resulted in over 75,000 fertility studies conducted between 1950 and 2000. Of these, only 381 dealt with fertility and reproduction behaviors involving males, two-thirds of which were biological and medical in orientation. These facts show that fertility theories and research have largely overlooked males. As Bledsoe and her associates (2000, p. 83) note, "men, if they appeared [in fertility] at all, usually did so as shadows; as partners-by-implication of those engaged in childbearing." Thus, Coleman (2000, p. 31) refers to males as "a neglected

L. Zhang, *Male Fertility Patterns and Determinants*, The Springer Series on Demographic Methods and Population Analysis 27, DOI 10.1007/978-90-481-8939-7_1,

minority" in fertility. Then why are men largely ignored in fertility studies? The next section of the chapter discusses several reasons to justify such exclusion.

1.1 Why Are Men Ignored in Fertility Studies?

To elucidate why men have been paid little attention in demographic and sociological studies of fertility, this section of the chapter discusses the biological, methodological, theoretical and sociological reasons. To begin with, the biological characteristics of females, namely puberty, menopause, and duration of pregnancy are sometimes viewed as reasons for choosing to focus on women when studying fertility (Hertrich, 1998). Compared to men, women have a more sharply defined and a narrower range (15–49) of reproductive years; and "both the spacing and number of children are less subject to variation among women: a woman can have children only at intervals of 1 or 2 years, whereas a man can have hundreds" (Keyfitz, 1977, p. 114). Put differently, women are more constrained by biological limitations, and hence are more influenced by the proximate determinants, say, by breastfeeding, than are males. In fact, several of the proximate determinants are virtually "man-free." In this sense, female fertility is considered as more fundamental than male fertility. Moreover, women are biologically directly involved in pregnancy and giving birth. Due to biological constraints, fertility of females is often studied by demographic and sociological literature. Measures of female fertility are usually used as main indicators of fertility as well.

Besides biological reasons, practical and methodological issues are also contributive to demographers' concentration on females. Historically, fertility data have been gathered mostly through interviewing women instead of men for many reasons. For instance, women are easier to be interviewed because previously they were more often at home than men. Women are also assumed to be able to provide proper information about their husbands' attitudes towards reproductive behavior (Shryock & Siegel, 1976). Additionally, data collected from women are considered more accurate than those collected from men because women are usually more directly involved in reproductive events, such as pregnancies and births (Courgeau, 1992; Hertrich, 1998; Poulain, Rianey, & Firdion, 1992). Even today, in most countries, data on parental age at the birth of the baby are more frequently gathered from the birth registration certificates for mothers than for fathers. This occurs because the indirect involvement of men in childbearing leads to a greater number of unreported ages for fathers, particularly for births occurring outside of marriage and among younger age groups (Poston & Chang, 2005). Data of infancy death are often gathered from women as well since men are found to be more likely to omit or overlook infant deaths (Hertrich, 1998; Seltzer, 1973). This is especially the case in some less industrialized regions, such as Africa, where levels of infant and child mortality rates are high. Considering these situations, more detailed questions for men are usually avoided in national surveys or censuses in many countries, making it more difficult to study fertility of men.

In addition to these practical matters, there are some methodological difficulties that have resulted in downplaying of men in fertility. Take classical demographic models as an example. These models are constructed as one-sex models, which only include females and leave males out. The stable population model, for instance, only takes age-specific fertility rates (ASFRs) and age-specific death rates (ASDRs) of females into consideration. Men are not included in demographic models because including men in these models requires generalizing the demographic events to men and taking into account the role of men in reproduction and population change. This generalization, however, is not easy, not only technically but also conceptually since it makes demographic models too complicated to be constructed (Pollak, 1986; Schoen, 1981). Methodological difficulties of including males in fertility models also exist in modeling fertility determinants for both sexes. It has been pointed out that demographic techniques are not sophisticated enough to "separate male and female factors affecting fertility" (Wood, 1994, p. 475). This is because variables that impact husband's and wife's fertility behaviors are usually intertwining with each other. Incorporating fertility determinants for both men and women into a single quantitative model is very difficult. From this perspective, Wood (1994, p. 17) contends that the existing single-sex and female-dominated tradition of fertility studies is largely "a matter of convenience . . . [because] the two-sex models of population dynamics are very much more complicated mathematically than single-sex models."

The exclusion of men does not only result from the above biological, practical and methodological realities of fertility, but also stems from the theoretical tradition of demography. Demographic theories explaining the fertility transition rarely require an involvement of men. As indicated earlier, the most popular explanatory theory of fertility, such as the proximate determinants theory, emphasizes factors such as marriage, contraceptive use and prevalence; but it does not necessarily demand data for both men and women (Greene & Biddlecom, 2000). The cost and benefit theory stresses the importance of rational calculation in reducing fertility, but it does not consider whether or not the value of children for men is also changing over time. The wealth flows perspective reveals the mechanism of fertility decline when a society transforms from a traditional patriarchal system to a more modernized system. The perspective, nevertheless, does not acknowledge the changing roles of males who are assumed to be the gatekeepers of conventional patriarchal social structure. This "lack of coherent theoretical grounding" in demography has somehow contributed to the unawareness of men in fertility (Greene & Biddlecom, 2000, p. 84).

Sociologically, men are often considered as less involved in fertility for they are regarded principally as breadwinners and "as typically uninvolved in fertility except to impregnate women and to stand in the way of their contraceptive use" (Greene & Biddlecom, 2000, p. 83). The traditional understanding of men's and women's roles is frequently described as "men work outside the home, whereas women are responsible for activities associated with the production of children and domestic services" (Watkins, 1993, p. 561). Even today, although the terms of gender and gender equity are gaining popularity, "gender" by and large is still more often considered a biological category than a sociological classification. The assumption of "consonance between men's and women's interests within marriage" has further played a part to the one-sex research interest in fertility studies (Greene & Biddlecom, 2000, p. 83). It is also a fact that children are more likely to be living with their mothers than with their fathers, especially in divorced families and when childbearing occurs in nonmarital unions (Shryock & Siegel, 1976). These facts have strengthened the belief that women are more closely tied to childbearing and childrearing than men. All of the factors discussed above have presented a social context for not considering men and men's role in fertility.

1.2 Male Fertility: An Important Component of Fertility Studies

Biology, nevertheless, dictates that females and males must both intimately be involved in the production of children. Fertility is not a process that only involves women. The male sex as a whole has an equivalent amount of contribution to reproduction as the female counterpart. In fact, the variation of each individual male's contribution to generating offspring is even considered as significantly greater than that of female. As it is observed that in most sexually reproducing mammalian species, "while most females reproduce, some males do not reproduce at all while others produce very large numbers of offspring" (Coleman, 2000, p. 33). This phenomenon is partially due to the sexual competition in the evolutionary process.

In demography, men's special features in fertility have also been demonstrated in several aspects. Paget and Timaeus (1994) show that male age-specific fertility has a later starting and much later stopping pattern as compared to female age-specific fertility. The median age of first births for men is found to be higher than that for women. In Norwegian countries, for example, the median ages of first births were 26 years and 23 years for men and women respectively in 1972; in Denmark in 1993, the median age was 31 for males and 28 for females (Coleman, 2000, p. 51). The effects of age on male and female fertility are revealed to be very different as well. Women reach their fertility peak between ages 25 and 35, at which time they begin to have a declining fertility until menopause. Men's reproductive ages, on the other hand, are in a gradual process which continue until death (Wood, 1994). When the cumulative pattern of fertility is considered, male total fertility rates (TFRs) are found to be different from those of females. It is shown that male TFRs were first higher than female TFRs in most Western industrialized countries before the 1960s. Such male and female fertility differentials are likely to be resulted from the relative shortage of men caused by two world wars. Since the 1960s, males in most industrialized countries have recovered from war time losses. Coupled with an increasing emigration that has been replaced by immigration which is largely dominated by men, male TFRs turned to be higher than female TFRs afterwards (Coleman, 2000). In addition to male and female fertility differentials in rates, demographers have also indicated that the progeny size distribution and childlessness patterns of men and women differentiate male fertility from female fertility. Some research shows that, in general, males are more likely to have a fewer number of children than females. Consequently, there are higher percentages of childless men as compared to women (Coleman, 2000).

All these facts suggest that human fertility cannot be fully represented by female fertility. Using female fertility rates to stand for male fertility rates can be problematic, especially in societies where divorce, remarrying and migration rates are fairly high. Researchers suggest that even applying marital female fertility rates to represent human fertility as an alternative solution is unsuitable because nonmarital birth rates in some societies are comparatively high and men are more likely to remarry than women after divorce, which makes male and female fertility not comparable (Greene & Biddlecom, 2000; Juby & Bourdais, 1998; Magnani, Bertrand, Makani, & McDonald, 1995). If fertility researchers are interested in taking a step further from examining fertility levels to fertility determinants, then involving men in fertility studies appears to be necessary as well. This is because childbearing is a process that includes couples' communication and negotiation. As the feminist thought argues, fertility research should study "the sexes in contrast with each other, not just the analysis of women's characteristics as determinants of fertility" (Greene & Biddlecom, 2000, p. 87). Only relying on females' responses to study human fertility determinants may bias the research results since women may not be able to provide reliable reports about their partners' social and economic background, their reproduction-related attitudes and behaviors. This situation is "most common among less-educated women, young women and those with larger numbers of births [as well as unmarried women]" (Goldscheider & Kaufman, 1996, p. 93).

Beyond investigating fertility determinants, examining other dimensions of fertility needs involving males as well. For example, understanding the timing of parenthood demands exploring closely the meaning of fatherhood and motherhood in various cultural institutions and how the meaning changes over the life course for men as compared to for women. Looking into the link between the construction and deconstruction of a childbearing and childrearing union (such as cohabitation and marriage) also requires knowing more about men's commitment in these unions. The women's health movement has also stressed the need for men to be aware of their responsibilities in family planning and reproductive health. In sum, it is imperative to bringing men into fertility and fertility-related research. Male fertility should be considered as an important component of fertility studies.

1.3 A Growing Body of Literature on Male Fertility

Acknowledging the importance of men in fertility studies coupled with the availability of male fertility data, there have been an increasing number of studies involving males in their analyses since the 1990s. Articles, book chapters and books on male fertility have begun to appear in the demographic literature.

In 1998, the journal *Demography* published a special issue, "Men in Families," which focused on men's involvement in parenting in the United States and men's reproductive behavior and parenting outside the United States. In 1996 and 2000, two major papers appeared in the journal *Population and Development Review* (Goldscheider & Kaufman, 1996; Greene & Biddlecom, 2000) that stressed the importance of involving men in fertility studies and suggested directions for future research on male reproductive roles. In 2000, *Fertility and the Male Life-Cycle in the Era of Fertility Decline* (Bledsoe, Guyer, & Lerner, 2000), a book based on the papers presented at a 1995 conference of the IUSSP was published. Another two major books examining male fertility also appeared since the 1990s: *Dynamics of Human Reproduction* by James W. Wood, Aldine De Gruyter Press (Wood, 1994) and *Transitions to Adulthood in Europe*, edited by Martine Corijn and Eric Klijzing, Kluwer Academic Publishers (Corijn & Klijzing, 2001).

Professional meetings of sociology and demography have also included male fertility studies in their sessions. At the American Sociological Association (ASA) 2006 Annual Meeting, two papers addressed patterns of male fertility and fatherhood in the Fertility and Reproduction Session (Hynes, Yang, Joyner, & Peters, 2006; Zhang, 2006). The Population Association of America (PAA) 2006 Annual Meeting included papers which addressed male reproduction and evaluated the quality of fertility data collected from men (Dribe & Stanfors, 2006; Guzzo & Furstenberg, 2006; Rendall et al., 2006). Chapter 2 will review existing male fertility literature in a more detailed manner.

In sum, the emergence of these pioneer studies highlights that despite the female-dominated tradition, male fertility has been drawing an increasing amount of research attention recently in demography and sociology. The newly available male fertility data sets that aid the analysis of male fertility will be introduced in Chapter 3 which deals with data and methods. In the next sub-section of the book, I will discuss the objectives and the structure of this book.

1.4 Objectives and Structure of the Book

There are two main objectives of this book: (1) To enhance the knowledge of male fertility by exploring male fertility patterns measured by rates; and (2) To explore male fertility determines, which provides evidence to construct male fertility theories. Thus, the focus of this book goes beyond the emphasis of previous literature that aims to challenge the female-dominated tradition. Instead, the research concentrates on examining how male fertility differs from or similar to female fertility both in rates and in determinants.

In order to achieve these goals, the research takes a gendered perspective by contrasting male and female fertility rates and the manners in which a variety of factors influence male and female fertility. The term "male fertility" in this book is analogous to female fertility, which refers to the actual production of children by men. When contrasting male and female fertility determinants, I draw on several reliable national datasets that include a large number of covariates to determine factors that differentiate men's and women's fertility outcomes.

Chapters in this book are organized in three parts. Part I includes this Introduction and Overview chapter and another two chapters (Chapters 2 and 3) which reviews male fertility literature and introduces data and methods, respectively. Part II (Chapters 4 and 5) begins to examine male and female by analyzing empirical data at the aggregate level. Chapter 4 examines male and female fertility rates in 43 countries and places. Chapter 5 focuses the analysis on a specific locale, namely, Taiwan, during 1949–2002. Part III shifts the research focus to fertility determinants of men and women at the individual level. Factors that have been found influential on female fertility are examined in this part and are treated in separate chapters, as well as integrated with other factors in particular chapters in this book. In each separate chapter, I compare the effects of the fertility determinants on male and on female fertility outcomes. In Chapter 6, I examine how demographic and socioeconomic factors differentiate men's and women's fertility. Chapter 7 deals with the effects of religion and religiosity on male fertility change as compared to female fertility variation. Chapter 8 and 9 investigate how cohabitation experience and cultural inheritance affect men's and women's fertility, respectively. Chapter 10 concludes findings and tries to bring together several areas of the book to elucidate how this book improves our understanding of male fertility and helps to construct male fertility theories. The final chapter also discusses the findings in light of future family planning policy actions. The ending remarks further place future research attention on taking men's roles into account when considering factors leading to decisions about bearing and rearing children.

References

Bledsoe, C., Guyer, J., & Lerner, S. (2000). *Fertility and male life-cycle in the era of fertility decline*. New York: Oxford University Press.

Bledsoe, C., Guyer, J. I., & Lerner, S. (2000). Introduction. In C. Bledsoe, J. I. Guyer, & S. Lerner (Eds.), *Fertility and male life-cycle in the era of fertility decline* (pp. 1–26). New York: Oxford University Press.

Bongaarts, J. (1994). The impact of the proximate determinants of fertility: A comment on reinis. *Population Studies*, *48*(1), 159–160.

Caldwell, J. C. (1982). *Theories of fertility decline*. London: Academic Press.

Coleman, D. A. (2000). Male fertility trends in industrial countries: Theories in search of some evidence. In C. Bledsoe, J. I. Guyer, & S. Lerner (Eds.), *Fertility and male life-cycle in the era of fertility decline* (pp. 29–60). New York: Oxford University Press.

Corijn, M., & Klijzing, E. (2001). *Transitions to adulthood in Europe*. New York: Kluwer Academic Publishers.

Courgeau, D. (1992). Impact of response errors on event history analysis. *Population: An English Selection*, *4*, 97–110.

Dribe, M., & Stanfors, M. A. (2006). *Education, work, and parenthood: The experience of young men and women in post-war Sweden*. California: Paper presented at the Population Association of America (PAA) Annual Meeting, Los Angeles.

Goldscheider, F. K., & Kaufman, G. (1996). Fertility and commitment: Bringing men back in. *Population and Development Review*, *22*(Supplement: Fertility in the United States" New Patterns, New Theories), 87–99.

Greene, M. E., & Biddlecom, A. E. (2000). Absent and problematic men: Demographic accounts of male reproductive roles. *Population and Development Review*, *26*(1), 81–115.

Greenhalgh, S. (1990). Toward a political economy of fertility: Anthropological contributions. *Population and Development Review*, *16*(1), 85–106.
Guzzo, K. B., & Furstenberg, F. F. J. (2006). Paper presented at the population association of America (PAA) annual meeting, Los Angeles, California.
Hertrich, V. (1998). Are men's and women's answers to be equally trusted? A dual collection of birth and marriage histories in a population in Mali. *Population: An English Selection*, *10*(2), 303–318.
Hynes, K., Yang, F. T. -A., Joyner, K., & Peters, H. E. (2006). *The transition to early fatherhood: National estimates based on multiple surveys*. Montreal: Paper presented at the American Sociological Association (ASA) Annual Meeting.
Juby, H., & Bourdais, C. L. (1998). The changing context of fatherhood in Canada: A life course analysis. *Population Studies*, *52*(2), 163–175.
Keyfitz, N. (1977). *Applied mathematical demography*. New York: Wiley.
Magnani, R. J., Bertrand, J. T., Makani, B., & McDonald, S. W. (1995). Men, marriage and fatherhood in Kinshasa, Zaire. *International Family Planning Perspectives*, *21*(1), 19–25.
Morgan, S. P., & Hagewen, K. J. (2005). Fertility. In D. L. J. Poston & M. Micklin (Eds.), *Handbook of population* (pp. 229–251). New York: Springer.
Notestein, F. W. (1953). *Economic problems of population change proceedings of the eighth international conference of agricultural Economists*. New York: Oxford University Press.
Paget, W. J., & Timaeus, I. M. (1994). A relational Gompertz model of male fertility: Development and assessment. *Population Studies*, *48*(2), 333–340.
Pollak, R. A. (1986). A reformulation of the two-sex problem. *Demography*, *23*(2), 247–259.
Poston, D. L. J., & Chang, C. -F. (2005). Bringing males in: A critical demographic plea for incorporating males in methodological and theoretical analyses of human fertility. *Critical Demography*, *1*, 1–15.
Poston, D. L., & Frisbie, W. P. (2005). Ecological demography. In D. L. J. Poston & M. Micklin (Eds.), *Handbook of population* (pp. 601–624). New York: Springer.
Poulain, M., Rianey, B., & Firdion, J. -M. (1992). Data from a life history survey and the Belgian population register: A comparison. *Population: An English Selection*, *4*, 77–96.
Rendall, M. S., Joyner, K., Peters, H. E., Yang, F., Handcock, M. S., & Ryan, A. (2006). *A Bayesian approach to combining population and survey data for male fertility estimation*. Los Angeles: Paper presented at the Annual Meetings of Population Association of America.
Schoen, R. (1981). The harmonic mean as the basis of a realistic two-sex marriage model. *Demography*, *18*(2), 201–216.
Seltzer, W. (1973). *Demographic data collection: A summary of experience*. New York: The Population Council.
Shryock, H. S., & Siegel, J. S. (1976). *The methods and materials of demography*. San Diego: Academic Press.
Watkins, S. C. (1991). *From provinces into nations: Demographic integration in Western Europe, 1870–1960*. New Jersey: Princeton University Press.
Watkins, S. C. (1993). If all we know about women was what we read in *demography*, what should we know? *Demography*, *30*(4), 551–577.
Wood, J. W. (1994). *Dynamics of human reproduction: Biology, biometry and demography*. New York: Aldine De Gruyter.
Zhang, L. (2006). *Patterns of male and female fertility*. Paper presented at the American Sociological Association (ASA) Annual Meeting, Montreal, Canada.

Chapter 2
Review of Male Fertility Literature

Chapter 1 has briefly pointed out a growing body of literature on male fertility in recent decades. In this chapter, I will provide a more in-depth review of literature on this topic, particularly in the fields of demography and sociology. I evaluate the merits, limitations and problematic issues associated with previous studies of male fertility. I also discuss the way in which this book fills the voids of prior literature.

The suggestion has been made that the majority of studies on male fertility are biological and medical in orientation (Poston & Chang, 2005). These biological or medical oriented studies of male fertility have covered the following major topics: (1) biological, behavioral and natural factors influencing male reproduction and reproductive health, such as cadmium, spermatogenesis, tripterygium hypglaucum, Ramadhan fast, smoking and temperature (Abbas & Basalamah, 1986; Archibong & Hills, 2000; Bujan & Mieusset, 1996; McLachlan, Newbold, Burow, & Li, 2001; Raji, Oloyo, & Morakinyo, 2006; Rispin, 2002); (2) contraceptive approaches regulating male fertility, including hydroxyurea, goyssypol, testosterone, injections, hormonal methods and immunological approaches (Archibong, Powell, & Hills, 2000; Frich, 1994; Handelsman, 2000; Talwar & Pal, 1994; Yu & Chan, 1998); and (3) diseases causing male infertility and sterility, for instance, Chlamydia trachomatis, Chlamydial Serology and other age-related diseases (Autoux, De Mouy, & Acar, 1987; Gdoura, Keskes-Ammar, Bouzid, Eb, & Orfila, 2001; Pflieger-Bruss, Schuppe, & Schill, 2004; Rolf, Kenkel, & Nieschlag, 2002; Sherr & Barry, 2004). Such biological and medical oriented studies account for more than two thirds of the existing male fertility literature. In the following sections of this chapter, I will focus on discussing some main topics covered by demographic or sociological studies of male fertility, followed by an evaluation of these analyses.

2.1 Men's Participation in Fertility Decision-Making and Family Planning

Assessing men's role in childbearing and their participation in family planning is an important topic that has been examined in many demographic studies of male

L. Zhang, *Male Fertility Patterns and Determinants*, The Springer Series on Demographic Methods and Population Analysis 27, DOI 10.1007/978-90-481-8939-7_2,

fertility. Using data from the Demographic and Health Surveys (DHS), researchers have examined men's role in fertility reduction and family planning in a number of less developed nations, especially in Africa (Lamptey, Nicholas, Ofosu-Amaah, & Lourie, 1978; Maharaj, 2001; Petro-Nustas, 1999). Results show that men in these less developed countries have an increasing knowledge of contraceptive use. They are highly involved in family planning and play a decisive role in childbearing decision-making. Research shows that in some African countries, such as Ghana, Kenya, Nigeria, Sudan and Zambia, where traditions of male-dominance and patrilineal family structures are strong, husbands' reproductive motivations and preferences greatly influence those of their wives. Men often decide whether a couple uses family planning methods and how many children a couple should have (DeRose & Ezeh, 2005; Dodoo, 1998; Isiugo-Abanihe, 1994; Khalifa, 1988; Lamptey et al., 1978; Mbizvo & Adamchak, 1991). In other words, men's motivations of contraceptive use and their fertility preferences eclipse those of their wives. In these populations, men are revealed to determine the pattern of *achieved* fertility to a large extent.

Additional evidence also reveals that though in some societies men basically make childbearing decisions, husbands' and wives' responses to *prospective* fertility can vary significantly. For instance, in Mott and Mott's (1985) research, they interview a number of selected couples in a village of Nigeria. They find that although husband's and wife's responses to family planning and *achieved* fertility in the population studied are similar, husband's and wife's responses to *prospective* fertility intentions are very different. On average, monogamous husbands want more additional children than their wives; but polygynous husbands want slightly fewer additional children than each of their wives (Mott & Mott, 1985). In a more recent study measuring the unmet needs of husbands and wives in three countries, Bangladesh, the Dominican Republic and Zambia, Becker (1999) also observes substantial differences between spouses in terms of contraceptive use and fertility intentions.

Given the decisive role of men in fertility decision-making and the differentials of husband's and wife's reproductive intensions revealed in some societies, researchers have proposed several possible strategies to advance family planning programs in less developed countries. Becker (1999); Odhiambo (1997) foster spousal communication and argue that the lack of communication between husbands and wives, rather than men's opposition to contraception, is the primary obstacle to family planning in some high fertility nations. Family planning programs in those places may focus on enhancing couples' communication to reduce fertility. Lundgren and colleagues (2005) use the case of El Salvador to emphasize the diffusion effect of informal networks among men and women on spreading family planning information in Africa. Through examining fertility decisions made by five generations of a South Indian family, Karaa, Stark, & Wolf (1997, p. 24) propose the importance of male motivation in regulating fertility. Karaa and associates (1997, p. 24) contend that "individual motivation rather than choice of methods is more important for positive male participation in family planning." One common feature of this group of analyses is that they all try to enhance family planning programs by emphasizing men's involvement and participation.

A few other studies shift their research focuses on men's role in fertility decision-making and family planning to more industrialized societies, such as the United States. Earlier research based on the U.S. samples has also documented a male-dominated pattern in determining childbearing in the early 1970s (Marciano, 1979). Later findings have begun to show greater gender equality in contraceptive use and childrearing decision-making processes (Grady, Tanfer, Billy, & Lincoln-Hanson, 1996). One study conducted by Sorenson (1989) points out that men's role in fertility and reproduction can be influenced by the interaction effects of various factors. Drawing samples from the Arizona, New Mexico and Texas Public Use Microdata Samples (PUMS), Sorenson (1989) finds that ethnic stereotypes and wives' educational attainments interact with each other to affect men's role in childbearing decision-making. Sorenson contends that non-Hispanic husbands have less of an effect on their wives' fertility behaviors when compared to Mexican-American couples. After controlling for differences in female educational attainments, however, the effect of ethnicity disappears. The author therefore argues that researchers should be cautious when studying fertility of population with a wide range of educational levels since the interaction effects may exist to influence men's role in fertility decision-making. Findings of the above analyses based on the U.S. social context seem to suggest a less dominant role of men in making childbearing decisions. In societies with greater gender equality such as the United States, men's role in fertility decision-making is likely to be affected by the interaction effects of a variety of demographic and socioeconomic factors.

2.2 Comparative Analyses of Male and Female Fertility Patterns and Determinants

Comparing patterns and determinants of male fertility with those of females is also a major topic discussed in previous studies of male fertility. Prior studies have examined age-specific and completed fertility patterns for both sexes and compared the determinants of male and female fertility. A few studies have also discussed factors that impact the timing of paternity and maternity and how timing of paternity impacts men's life-cycle.

In regard to the age pattern of fertility, as many other fertility measures, greater attention has been paid to females. Researchers propose the following reasons to justify the concentration on maternity age: the effects of female age on fertility are strong; the age effect on couple's fertility rates is largely attributed to female age; and there is a lack of knowledge about the impact of biological factors on male fecundity (Anderson, 1975; Smith, 1972). More available data on maternal age than on paternal age also makes measuring female age-specific fertility easier than male fertility.

Despite more research attention to female-age specific fertility, a few studies have examined the effect of male age on fertility and the age-specific pattern of male reproduction. Anderson (1975) finds that fertility can be considerably affected by male age, particularly in non-contraceptive populations, such as population of

Ireland in the early 1900s. Paget and Timaeus (1994) also observe that male age-specific fertility pattern differs from that of their female counterparts. It has a pattern of starting later, having a later and lower peak, and remaining higher than that of females with increasing age. Kiernan and Diamond's (1983) study of the British cohort of 1946 echo the results of Paget and Timaeus and show that men tend to have their first births later compared to women (a median age of 25.9 for men versus 23.0 for women). Also, the first birth distribution of males appears to be more dispersed than that of females. By exploring the age-specific fertility pattern of the U.S. men in a detailed manner, Thomas' (1996) research echoes results of previous literature and illustrates the special features of male age-specific fertility as compared to that of females.

In addition to the age-specific fertility differentials by sex, the male and female fertility differentials are also exhibited in comparative analyses of completed fertility for both sexes. Kuczynski (1932) calculates male and female net reproduction rates (NRRs) in France during 1920–1923 and shows that male and female NRRs were far from identical (1.19 and 0.98, respectively). The male and female difference in NRRs is considered to be caused by the shortage of men as a result of World War I. Coleman (2000) also notes that since the 1960s, male completed fertility rates have been lower than those of females in most European nations. For example, the TFRs in France in 1974 were 2.05 for males and 2.11 for females; in Denmark in 1988, the TFRs were 1.37 and 1.50 for males and females, respectively. Male and female fertility dynamics in the United States have shown a similar pattern as those in European countries indicated by Coleman. That is, male completed fertility began to be lower than that of females in recent years. As Ventura, Martin, Curtin, Matthews, & Park (2000) show, male TFR was higher than female TFR in 1980 (1.97 for males versus 1.84 for females). In 1992, however, the reverse pattern became true considering the TFRs for U.S. men and women were 2.05 and 2.11, respectively (2000). Since then, male TFRs continued to be lower than those of females in the U.S. In 2000, for instance, male and female TFRs were 2.02 and 2.06, respectively. In Taiwan, Zhang and colleagues (Zhang, Poston, & Chang, 2010) also find that male TFRs used to be higher than female TFR. They then had a crossover in the late 1980s and female fertility rates began to be higher than male TFRs afterwards. These findings suggest that male and female fertility differentials do exist in various societies. The general pattern seems to be that male fertility used to be higher than female fertility and the reverse pattern is true in recent years.

Recognizing the age-specific and total fertility differentials by gender, scholars have expanded their research interests to male fertility determinants and factors that differentiate male and female fertility. As far as male fertility determinants, Harter (1968) exhibits that motivation for contraceptive use can a better predictor of male excess fertility than knowledge of contraception or behavioral involvement, controlling for education, race and ethnicity and religious participation. Through studying the number of children 16,777 American men have fathered, Bachu (1996) shows that Hispanic origin, socioeconomic status and nationality influence marital fertility of American men. In general, Hispanic origin with lower socioeconomic status increases the number of children ever born (CEB) reported by men. When both the husband and wife are foreign born, the male fertility rates tend to be higher than if both spouses are native born. In terms of factors that differentiate men's and women's fertility, Bachu finds that for never-married population, some demographic factors such as nationality, race and ethnicity have different influences on fertility for men when compared to their effects on women. To illustrate, foreign-born men are more likely to be childless than foreign-born women. Never-married Black women report having an average of 1.2 births; while never-married Black men report an average CEB of 0.5. In addition, Bachu (1996) demonstrates that the effect of marital status on fertility varies by gender. Fertility rates of never-married men are considerably lower than fertility of never-married women.

Besides investigating fertility determinants, some recent studies have analyzed survey data from twenty-four European countries for the 1980s and 1990s to study socioeconomic factors that impact paternity and maternity. The results show that the general negative effect of educational attainment on entering into parenthood is stronger for women than for men. Unemployment leads to men's postponement of marriage and having children, whereas it affects women in two distinct ways. It either accelerates or slows down women's timing of marriage and having children. The effect of religion on childbearing is stronger among women than men. Further, being Catholic and attending church services affect men's and women's parenthood timing in different ways in predominantly Catholic countries (Corijn & Klijzing, 2001).

Male fertility related issues, such as the timing of paternity, are also examined as independent variables to show their effects on men's life-cycle events. Results show that males with early first birth occurrences tend to have shorter educational attainment and income trajectories. Men who are teenage fathers are less likely to pursue higher education and more likely to earn less than men who defer parenthood (Pirog-Good & Good, 1995; Thomas, 1996). Moreover, males who experience an early age at first birth are less "able and willing" to be fathers since paternity is intimately related to the obligation of financially supporting the children (Thomas, 1996, p. 2). However, males who defer fatherhood are found to be more involved and highly affective with their children (Cooney, Pedersen, Indelicato, & Palkovitz, 1993).

2.3 Modeling Male Fertility and Constructing Two-Sex Models

In addition to the two major topics discussed above, modeling male fertility and constructing two-sex models is the third major concern of previous demographic studies on male fertility. As Pollak (1986, p. 400) states, the classical stable population theory is a "one-sex" theory, that is, only female matters. Pollak argues that age-specific fertility schedules and age-specific mortality schedules of females are the two building blocks of the classical stable population theory. In fact, not only the stable population theory but many other demographic models have excluded men in the analysis. To challenge the one-sex tradition of model constructing, efforts have been made to reconcile male and female rates in the analyses of stable populations date back at least to the work of Karmel (1947). Following Karmel, demographers have attempted to introduce male paternity and mortality schedules into the classic models (Coale, 1972; Kuhn, 1978). Some researchers also recommend incorporating age composition of men and women into demographic models since they find there are gender interaction effects on childbearing, which is resulted from the available numbers of men and women in the marriage market. Such effects are often referred to as birth function and marriage function (Das Gupta, 1973; 1978; McFarland, 1975; Mitra, 1976; 1978; Schoen, 1977; 1981).

Beyond the effort made to incorporate males in conventional demographic models, researchers have also tried to build male fertility models to reflect male fertility dynamics. Using data from the United Nations *Demographic Yearbook*, Paget and Timaeus (1994) propose a male fertility standard by applying the female standards to males to represent male fertility variation. The traditional two-step transformation of Booth's female standard can only be used to represent male fertility patterns in high fertility countries. The two-parameter relational Gompertz fertility model that is based on the standard Paget and Timaeus have proposed can represent male fertility distributions in a variety of countries. This is a significant contribution to male fertility modeling.

2.4 An Evaluation of Prior Literature

Previous demographic and sociological studies of male fertility discussed above have focused on addressing men's role in fertility decision-making, the male and female fertility differentials in rates and in determinants, and issues related to constructing two-sex demographic models. These studies have considerably advanced our understanding of male fertility. The association explored between the age pattern of reproduction and other life events of men underscores the magnitude of men in reproduction, family formation and childrearing. Moreover, the fertility differentials by gender revealed by previous studies have called attention to bringing men into fertility studies because female fertility cannot fully represent human fertility. As Poston and Chang (Poston & Chang, 2005, p. 15) argue, "demographers and sociologists should give more attention to males in their analyses of fertility variation and change than has heretofore been the case. . .it is no longer acceptable or appropriate to estimate fertility models that are based solely on women and on female fertility rates." The reviewed studies, in general, have challenged the status quo of conventional demography that concentrates exclusively on female fertility and have emphasized the importance of studying men in fertility and fertility-related events.

Important policy implications may be drawn from the reviewed work as well. Many previous family planning policies have principally been geared towards educating women and stressed women's role in contraceptive use and family planning. Increasing women's labor force participation and educational attainments are considered as key means of lowering fertility in many countries (Rindfuss, Morgan, &

Offutt, 1996; Smith-Lovin & Tickamyer, 1978). This group of work, on the other hand, emphasizes men's role in childbearing decision-making. Researchers suggest that men should be the target of family planning programs, particularly in societies with a patriarchal structure. In those societies, without the involvement of men in family planning, policies merely involve females may well be futile. Previous studies make the point clearly that while relying on informal networks, spousal communication and increasing women's reproductive autonomy in facilitating transition of fertility to a lower level, men's responsibility in childbearing should also be taken into consideration.

As far as the attempt of constructing two-sex models, including men in fertility models makes significant contributions to demographic modeling. Lotka's (1911) stable population theory, for example, is only concerned with how female birth and death patterns influence overall population change. If Lotka's theory was applied to male and female populations separately, it would lead to two different intrinsic growth rates for two sexes. This feature constrains the applicability of the stable population theory. Including men in demographic models, as Gupta (1978) argues, helps to obtain a single rate of intrinsic growth that combines male and female birth and death rates together. This combination reconciles the male-female conflict in the stable population theory by generating intrinsic age-specific fertility rates and intrinsic net reproduction rates for males and females. These rates are consistent and can operate simultaneously on a population. As such, the two-sex modeling approach is able to remove the limitation in Lotka's stable-population theory. It may also be used to improve other classical demographic models. The two-sex modeling strategy may provide possible directions for future modeling paths as well.

An additional contribution of including men in demographic models is that the two-sex models illustrate the substance of a population's age-sex structure and the gender interaction effects when studying fertility. The two-sex models seek to find a mathematical expression that depicts how men and women interact with respect to their relative ages. The birth function presented in these models "reflects the age pattern of the male-female interaction as of the base year" (Gupta, 1978, p. 368). The marriage function considered by demographers who construct two-sex models takes male-female age pattern and timing and, in addition, male and female nuptiality-mortality life table into consideration when determining fertility (Gupta, 1978; McFarland, 1975; Schoen, 1977). These two functions well demonstrate that the gender interactions are essential components of demographic modeling of fertility. Such interaction effects should be included in demographic analyses and will lead to meaningful implications for male fertility studies. These concerns would have not been addressed if males were excluded from the analysis. Paget and Timaeus's (1994) work makes a contribution to male fertility modeling by generating male standards based on female standards, which is initiative and will have profound impacts on future modeling strategies of male fertility.

In spite of the strengths of previous studies, there are also some limitations. The first inadequacy lies in the manner in which male fertility is calculated when comparing male and female fertility rates. The idea of applying female fertility measures to males is sound, while some of the measures used to represent male fertility in prior analyses are questionable. One common technique calculating male fertility in existing studies is to apply the number of children to women in a certain year divided by the mid-year male population. This approach is appropriate when computing the general fertility rate (GFR), the crude birth rate (CBR) and other rates that do not need to consider the age effects on fertility. However, when the age effects on fertility are taken into account, this approach can be problematic because the assumption behind this technique is that men and women have an equal amount of children in a particular age group during a specific time period. This assumption is actually not true in most populations. In reality, females tend to have more births in younger ages than males and the opposite situation is the case for older ages (this fact will be highlighted in Chapter 4 that studies male and female fertility in Taiwan). Thus, using the same numerators (number of births given by females) to generate male age-specific fertility rates (ASFRs) and total fertility rates (TFRs) is not appropriate. The results based on analyzing these male fertility rates may need to be reassessed.

The second flaw of previous analyses regards the issues that explain the changing pattern of male and female fertility. This flaw may result from the way in which male fertility is calculated as discussed above. Coleman (2000) notes that the changing pattern of male and female fertility differentials in rates can be interpreted by the existence of unequal numbers of males and females in various time periods. From the nineteenth century to the 1950s, emigration, military services and warfare led to a shortage of males, which generated a higher proportion of never-married females in Western societies from the early nineteenth century until the mid twentieth century. Thus, male fertility rates were higher than female fertility rates during this time frame. After World War II, the recovery of the male population from wartime losses and emigration replaced by immigration that is dominated by males in most industrialized counties have resulted in relatively more males in each age cohort than females. Coleman therefore contends that this is the reason why male TFRs became slightly lower than those of females.

Such an explanation is based on fertility changes caused by denominators. As discussed above, if the approach used to compute male fertility rates is questionable, then the explanations of male and female fertility differentials based upon such a rationale would need to be re-examined. Even if the shortage of men caused by two world wars is a possible reason that has resulted in fertility differences by gender in some European countries, this account may not be applicable to other societies. For instance, almost four decades following WWII, until 1990, male TFRs were still higher than female TFRs in the United States and in Taiwan. So the explanation relying on the relative sizes of male and female population affected by two world wars is not adequate to explain the male and female fertility differentials in rates, especially in non-European regions. Exploring other reasons, especially in the social context of non-European countries is warranted.

Furthermore, male and female fertility differentials in rates shown in most prior studies are examined from a longitudinal point of view. The association between male and female fertility changes has rarely been examined cross-sectionally. Future research may improve current literature with regard to this aspect.

In terms of research on male fertility determinants, previous analyses have not systematically modeled the combined effects of demographic characteristics and socioeconomic variables on male completed fertility, such as CEB and TFR. Other important factors that have been found crucial to female fertility, such as cohabitation and religion, have not been applied to male fertility analyses after controlling for other factors. More importantly, fertility differentials shown in previous studies have rarely been statistically tested. Such differentials may be due to dissimilar male and female sample sizes or standard errors. Thus, a multivariate analysis that statistically tests the gender interaction effects is necessary to elucidate factors that differentiate men's and women's fertility.

Among studies of men's role in childbearing decision-making and family planning, one may have realized that much of the reviewed literature is based on less industrialized countries. This probably reflects researchers' greater concern for fertility reduction in high-fertility countries where declines in women's desired fertility does not necessarily lead to lower fertility (Goldscheider & Kaufman, 1996). Limited sources of male fertility data may be another reason that much less work has been done for highly industrialized nations. As one of the principal data sources that contain male fertility information, the DHS dataset, for example, mainly surveys populations of developing countries, such as countries in Africa and Asia. This may have led to the fact that the majority of the studies that examine men's participating in fertility-decision making focus on the African continent. Although a few studies present results based on analyzing the U.S. samples, it is not clear if the pattern of equally sharing childbearing responsibilities between husbands and wives is universal in other industrialized nations. Also, under the circumstance of gender equality, the communication and negotiation between men and women in other sexual unions, such as cohabitation unions, has not been explored in either developed or developing countries. The interaction effects of other socioeconomic factors with gender in determining childbearing are also worthy of exploration in future analyses.

Given the merits and shortcomings of these studies, in this book, I intend to improve male fertility studies by filling some voids of prior literature. As indicated in Chapter 1, two central aims under the gendered scope guide this current analysis. First, I explore the male and female fertility differentials in rates from both longitudinal and cross-sectional viewpoints. This fills the gap of previous research that merely studies male and female fertility differentials in rates from a longitudinal point of view. I rely on data released by the United Nations *Demographic Yearbook* to study male and female TFRs in 43 countries and places cross-sectionally during 1990–1998. When studying male and female fertility differentials in rates, I expand the focuses of previous research on male fertility from the European continent and African countries to an Eastern society, namely, Taiwan. Datasets available for this particular locale allow me to contrast male and female fertility rates in this region for several decades longitudinally, and in 23 counties of Taiwan in a specific year cross-sectionally. A unique feature of the Taiwan analysis is that male fertility is calculated in a more accurate manner than previous studies. The male fertility rates are generated by number of children by males in a specific age group divided by number of males in the same age group. This approach avoids the measurement errors that may appear in previous studies as noted above.

The analysis of male fertility in Taiwan also provides additional answers to explicate why male and female fertility differs in rates. I show that educational attainment can be a factor that explains male and female fertility differentials by age. I also propose that the issue of mate availability could be a reason that differentiates men's and women's fertility outcomes. Previous studies have shown that mate availability in the marriage market is strongly related to the level of fertility. An abundance of eligible males in the local marriage market is found to increase the rate of women entering into marriage and the risk of nonmarital childbearing (Fossett & Kiecolt, 1993; South, 1996; South & Lloyd, 1992). In Taiwan, due to the tradition of preferencing a male heir, there are now a large number of extra boys born each year than girls (Hudson & den Boer, 2004; Poston, Dudley, & Zhang, 2007; Tucker et al., 2005). Consequently, there are a greater number of males available in the marriage market than females. Such a situation may lead to the female marital rate being higher than that of males. Thus, I propose that the relatively higher female marital rate resulting from the unbalanced sex ratios at birth (SRB) may be a cause of higher female than male fertility in Taiwan. Unlike previous studies that explain male and female fertility differentiation from the perspective of the shortage of men caused by two world wars, my analysis takes educational factor and cultural tradition into consideration to investigate fertility differentiation by gender. These studies will enrich current analyses on male and female fertility trends and patterns measured by various fertility rates.

The second aim of this book is to scrutinize male fertility determinants as compared to female fertility determinants in a more comprehensive manner by analyzing the U.S. samples. When I conceptualize the factors that may have an impact on male fertility, I consider factors that span demographic, social, economic, cultural, religious and biological aspects of existence. This broad research agenda is drawn from several popular demographic theories enlightening female fertility variation. This agenda helps to comprehend a great deal about factors influence men's fertility outcomes. Further, the book differentiates it from other discussions of factors associated with variation in male fertility by launching more sophisticated statistical techniques. Early work on male fertility determinants often employed fairly simple descriptive statistics or univariate statistics. It is hard to disentangle the partial effect of a particular factor on male fertility from many other covariates. In this research, I apply more advanced statistical methods to account for the impacts of a number of variables as they relate to male fertility variation, controlling for the effects of other covariates. I statistically test the gender interaction effects, which aims to exhibit how various factors influence men's and women's fertility in significantly different manners. By linking the aggregate and individual level analyses together, this book elaborates the trends and patterns of male as compared to those of females. It tells a story about how a variety of demographic and socioeconomic factors affect men's fertility.

2.5 Summary

To summarize, I review prior studies on male fertility and related issues in this chapter. Particular attention is given to demographic and sociological oriented research. Highlighting men's role in fertility decision-making and family planning, constructing two-sex fertility models, and comparatively examining fertility differentials by gender appear to be major topics covered by recent studies on male fertility. Strengths and limitations of prior literature are assessed at the end of the chapter, which points out directions for future research. In order to improve existing studies on male fertility, I outline two levels of analyses in this monograph to examine patterns and determinants of male fertility from a gendered perspective. Data and methods used to pursue the empirical work will be specified in the following chapter.

References

Abbas, S. M., & Basalamah, A. H. (1986). Effects of Ramadhan fast on male fertility. *Archives of Andrology, 16*(2), 161–166.

Anderson, B. A. (1975). Male age and fertility results from Ireland prior to 1911. *Population Index, 41*(4), 561–567.

Archibong, A. E., & Hills, E. R. (2000). Male fertility as affected by cadmium: Immunocontraceptive potential. *Advances in Reproduction, June 4*(2–3), 25–35.

Archibong, A. E., Powell, A., & Hills, E. R. (2000). Male fertility as affected by hydroxyures: Clinical application/contraceptive potential. *Advances in Reproduction, 4*(2–3), 3.

Autoux, M. R., De Mouy, D. M., & Acar, J. F. (1987). Male fertility and positive chlamydial serology: A study of 61 fertile and 82 subfertile men. *Journal of Andrology, 8*(3), 197–200.

Bachu, A. (1996). *Fertility of American men*: U.S. census bureau population division working paper, No. 14.

Becker, S. (1999). Measuring unmet need: Wives, husbands or couples? *International Family Planning Perspectives, 25*(4), 172–180.

Bujan, L., & Mieusset, R. (1996). Temperature and male fertility. *Contraception, Fertility and Sexualite, 24*(6), 429–438.

Coale, A. J. (1972). *The growth and structure of human populations: A mathematical investigation* Princeton, NJ: Princeton University Press.

Coleman, D. A. (2000). Male fertility trends in industrial countries: Theories in search of some evidence. In C. Bledsoe, J. I. Guyer, & S. Lerner (Eds.), *Fertility and male life-cycle in the era of fertility decline* (pp. 29–60). New York: Oxford University Press.

Cooney, T. M., Pedersen, F. A., Indelicato, S., & Palkovitz, R. (1993). Timing of fatherhood: Is "on-time" optimal? *Journal of Marriage and the Family, 55*(1), 205–215.

Corijn, M., & Klijzing, E. (2001). *Transitions to adulthood in Europe*: New York: Kluwer Academic Publishers.

Das Gupta, P. (1973). Growth of U.S. population, 1940–1971, in the light of an interactive two-sex model. *Demography, 10*(4), 543–565.

Das Gupta, P. (1978). An alternative formulation of the birth function in a two-sex model. *Population Studies, 32*(2), 367–379.

DeRose, L. F., & Ezeh, A. C. (2005). Men's influence on the onset and progress of fertility decline in Ghana, 1988–98. *Population Studies, 59*(2), 197–210.

Dodoo, F. N.-A. (1998). Men matter: Additive and interactive gendered preferences and reproductive behavior in Kenya. *Demography, 35*(2), 229–242.

Fossett, M. A., & Kiecolt, K. J. (1993). Mate availability and family structure among African Americans in U.S. metropolitan areas. *Journal of Marriage and the Family, 55*(2), 288–302.
Frich, J. (1994). The development of male contraceptives. *South to South Newsletter, 3*, 10–12.
Gdoura, R., Keskes-Ammar, F., Bouzid, F., Eb, A. H., & Orfila, J. (2001). Chlamydia trachomatis and male infertility in Tunisia. *The European Journal of Contraception and Reproductive Health, 6*(2), 102–107.
Goldscheider, F. K., & Kaufman, G. (1996). Fertility and commitment: Bringing men back in *Population and Development Review, 22*(Supplement: Fertility in the United States New Patterns, New Theories), 87–99.
Grady, W. R., Tanfer, K., Billy, J. O. G., & Lincoln-Hanson, J. (1996). Men's perceptions of their roles and responsibilities regarding sex, contraception and childrearing. *Family Planning Perspectives, 28*(5), 221–226.
Gupta, P. D. (1978). An alternative formulation of the birth function in a two-sex model. *Population Studies, 32*(2), 367–379.
Handelsman, D. J. (2000). Hormonal male contraception. *International Journal of Andrology, 23*(Suppl. 2), 8–12.
Harter, C. L. (1968). Male fertility in New Orleans. *Demography, 5*(1), 61–78.
Hudson, V. M., & den Boer, A. M. (2004). *Bare branches: The security implications of Asia's surplus male population*: Massachusetts: The MIT Press.
Isiugo-Abanihe, U. C. (1994). Reproductive motivation and family-size preferences among Nigerian men. *Studies in Family Planning, 25*(3), 149–161.
Karaa, M. V., Stark, N. N., & Wolf, J. (1997). Male involvement in family planning: A case study spanning five generations of a South Indian family. *Studies in Family Planning, 28*(1), 24–34.
Karmel, P. H. (1947). The relations between male and female reproduction rates. *Population Studies, 1*(3), 249–274.
Khalifa, M. A. (1988). Attitudes of Urban sudanese men toward family planning. *Studies in Family Planning, 19*(4), 236–243.
Kiernan, K. E., & Diamond, I. (1983). The age at which childbearing starts – a longitudinal study. *Population Studies, 37*(3), 363–380.
Kuczynski, R. R. (1932). *Fertility and reproduction*, Falcon Press, New York.
Kuhn, T. S. (1978). *The structure of scientific revolutions* (2nd edn.). Chicago: University of Chicago Press.
Lamptey, P., Nicholas, D. D., Ofosu-Amaah, S., & Lourie, I. M. (1978). An evaluation of male contraceptive acceptance in Rural Ghana. *Studies in Family Planning, 9*(8), 222–226.
Lundgren, R. I., Gribble, J. N., Greene, M. E., Emrick, G. E., & de Monroy, M. (2005). Cultivating men's interest in family planning in Rural El Salvador. *Studies in Family Planning, 36*(3), 173–188.
Maharaj, P. (2001). Male attitudes to family planning in the Era of HIV/AIDS: Evidence from KwaZulu-Natal, South Africa. *Journal of Southern African Studies, 27*(2), 245–257.
Marciano, T. D. (1979). Male influences on fertility: Needs for research. *The Family Coordinator, 28*(4), 561–568.
Mbizvo, M. T., & Adamchak, D. J. (1991). Family planning knowledge, attitudes, and practices of men in Zimbabwe. *Studies in Family Planning, 22*(1), 31–38.
McFarland, D. D. (1975). Models of marriage formation and fertility. *Social Forces, 54*(1), 66–83.
McLachlan, J. A., Newbold, R. R., Burow, M. E., & Li, S. F. (2001). From malformations to molecular mechanisms in the male: Three decades of research on Endocrine Disrupters. *APMIS, 109*, 263–272.
Mitra, S. (1976). Effect of adjustment for sex composition in the measurement of fertility on intrinsic rates. *Demography, 13*(2), 251–257.
Mitra, S. (1978). On the derivation of a two-sex population model. *Demography, 15*(4), 541–548.
Mott, F. L., & Mott, S. H. (1985). Household fertility decisions in West Africa: A comparison of male and female survey results. *Studies in Family Planning, 16*(2), 88–99.
Odhiambo, O. (1997). Men's participation in family planning decisions in Kenya. *Population Studies, 51*(1), 29–40.

Paget, W. J., & Timaeus, I. M. (1994). A relational Gompertz model of male fertility: Development and assessment. *Population Studies, 48*(2), 333–340.
Petro-Nustas, W. (1999). Men's knowledge of and attitudes toward birthspacing and contraceptive use in Jordan. *International Family Planning Perspectives, 25*(4), 181–185.
Pflieger-Bruss, S., Schuppe, H. C., & Schill, W. B. (2004). The male reproductive system and its susceptibility to endocrine disrupting chemicals. *Andrologia, 36*(6), 337–345.
Pirog-Good, M. A., & Good, D. H. (1995). Child support enforcement for teenage fathers: Problems and prospects. *Journal of Policy Analysis and Management, 14*(1), 25–42.
Pollak, R. A. (1986). A reformulation of the two-sex problem. *Demography, 23*(2), 247–259.
Poston, D. L. J., & Chang, C.-F. (2005). Bringing males in: A critical demographic plea for incorporating males in methodological and theoretical analyses of human fertility. *Critical Demography, 1*(1), 1–15.
Poston, J., Dudley L., & Zhang, L. (2007). How many extra boys have been born in China? In X. Zheng, D. L. J. Poston, & B. Gu (Eds.), *Gender and sexually transmitted infections in China*. Beijing: Peking University Press.
Raji, Y., Oloyo, A. K., & Morakinyo, A. O. (2006). Effect of methanol extrac of ricinus communis seed on reproduction of male rates. *Asian Journal of Andrology, 8*(1), 115–121.
Rindfuss, R. R., Morgan, P., & Offutt, K. (1996). Education and the changing age pattern of American fertility: 1963–1989. *Demography, 33*(3), 277–290.
Rispin, P. (2002). Occupational factors have little effect on male fertility. *Urology Times, 30*(2), 19.
Rolf, C., Kenkel, S., & Nieschlag, E. (2002). Age-related disease pattern in infertile men: Increasing incidence of infections in older patients. *Andrologia, 34*(4), 209–217.
Schoen, R. (1977). A two-sex nuptiality-mortality life table. *Demography, 14*(3), 333–350.
Schoen, R. (1981). The harmonic mean as the basis of a realistic two-sex marriage model. *Demography, 18*(2), 201–216.
Sharp, F. R., & Lotka, A. J. (1911). A problem in age-distribution. *Philosophical Magazine, 21*, 435–438.
Sherr, L., & Barry, N. (2004). Fatherhood and HIV-positive heterosexual men. *HIV Medicine, 5*(4), 258–263.
Smith, D. (1972). The demographic history of colonial New England. *Journal of Economic History, 32*, 165–183.
Smith-Lovin, L., & Tickamyer, A. R. (1978). Nonrecursive models of labor force participation, fertility behavior and sex role attitudes. *American Sociological Review, 43*(4), 541–557.
Sorenson, A. M. (1989). Husbands' and wives' characteristics and fertility decisions: A diagonal mobility model. *Demography, 26*(1), 125–135.
South, S. J. (1996). Mate availability and the transition to unwed motherhood: A paradox of population structure. *Journal of Marriage and the Family, 58*(2), 265–279.
South, S. J., & Lloyd, K. M. (1992). Marriage markets and nonmarital fertility in the United States. *Demography, 29*(2), 247–264.
Talwar, G. P., & Pal, R. (1994). Immunological control of male fertility. *Archives of Andrology, 7*(2), 177–185.
Thomas, V. S. (1996). *The age pattern of male fertility in the U.S. 1957–1964 birth cohorts*. Unpublished dissertation, Duke University, Durham, NC.
Tucker, J. D., Hendersona, G. E., Wang, T. F., Huang Y. Y., Parish W., Pan S. M., et al. (2005). Surplus men, sex work, and the spread of HIV in China. *AIDS, 19*(6), 539–547.
Ventura, S. J., Martin, J. A., Curtin, S. C., Matthews, T. J., & Park, M. M. (2000). *Births: Final Data for 1998*: National Vital Statistics Reports 48.
Yu, Z.-H., & Chan, H. C. (1998). Gossypol as a male antifertility agent – why studies should have been continued. *International Journal of Andrology, 21*(1), 2–7.
Zhang, L., Poston, J., Dudley L., & Chang, C.-F. (2010). Male and female fertility in Taiwan. In J. Poston, L. Dudley, & W. Yang (Eds.), *The family and social change in Chinese societies*. New York: Springer.

Chapter 3
Data and Methods

Since the results and conclusions of each analysis can be affected by data and research methodologies involved, I devote this chapter to an explication of the data and methods used throughout this study. Such discussion should enlighten the reader the data, methodological and statistical issues I have confronted and solved in the analysis. The chapter also addresses the data quality issue in male fertility reports that is raised by prior research. The detailed discussion on data and methods in this chapter should enable future research to both replicate and extend findings of this research.

3.1 Data

Dramatic improvements have taken place in the sources of data containing male fertility information. Although the majority of fertility surveys are still geared towards collecting fertility information of women, a number of data sources reporting men's fertility patterns have recently come into existence at the national level. These available data sources have resulted in major breakthroughs in the ability of researchers to specify detailed fertility models that include males. In this part of the chapter, I will explicate a number of newly available male fertility data sources, including those that will be analyzed in this study. All these datasets have special features regarding the nature and amount of male fertility information presented. Among the datasets introduced here, several of them allow comparison of male and female fertility in rates; others contain extremely detailed microlevel data for contrasting fertility determinants for both sexes. The following subsections will describe features of these datasets and their linkage for the purpose of analyzing male fertility in a variety of social contexts.

3.1.1 The United Nations Demographic Yearbook

The first data source that will be depicted here is the United Nations *Demographic Yearbook*. The *Demographic Yearbook* is one of the major demographic and

L. Zhang, *Male Fertility Patterns and Determinants*, The Springer Series on Demographic Methods and Population Analysis 27, DOI 10.1007/978-90-481-8939-7_3,

social statistics published by the United Nations. The statistical results released by the *Demographic Yearbook* are based on data collected from national statistical authorities since 1948 through a set of questionnaires dispatched annually by the United Nations Statistics Division to over 230 national statistical offices (http://unstats.un.orf/unsd/demographic/products/dyb/default.htm). The official statistics that been collected, compiled, and disseminated by the *Demographic Yearbook* focus on a wide range of topics. Major topics covered are: population size and composition, births, deaths, marriage and divorce. Statistics based on these topics are released to public on an annual basis. Beyond the above topics, some additional topics, such as economic activity, educational attainment, household characteristics, housing, ethnicity and languages have also been covered by special issues of the *Demographic Yearbook.*

The United Nations *Demographic Yearbook* is considered as one of the major data sources containing male fertility information because it presents birth rates by age of mothers and fathers in the issues of 1949–1950, 1954, 1959, 1965, 1969, 1975, 1981, 1986 and 1990–1998 (Coleman, 2000; United Nations, 2001). Birth rates in these issues are presented in the form of the ASFRs. Depending on various research interests, researchers may generate other measures of fertility based, such as TFRs, based on the ASFRs, to examine fertility patterns of men in a variety of countries. Comparative studies of male and female fertility by using this specific data source may be conducted at the national level as well.

I need to point out that though female fertility rates have been reported in a large number of countries, there are only a limited number of countries that have had male fertility rates available in the *Demographic Yearbook.* The lack of male fertility reports is especially common for illegitimate births in most countries. I have addressed a number of reasons in Chapter 1 why female fertility is considered as more fundamental than male fertility. Those reasons can probably explain why most countries do not report or even collect male fertility data in the *Demographic Yearbook.*

The reader should also be aware that for countries that have had both male and female fertility data available in the United Nations *Demographic Yearbook,* they are likely to be developed nations with relatively more advanced population registration systems. Some European countries, for example, fertility rates for both men and women reported in a number of years. Such a phenomenon perhaps suggests that some demographically or economically more advanced nations have already realized the importance of men in fertility and reproduction. Their more advanced population registration systems have also provided them the capability of bringing in men in natal registrations.

Given that fertility rates presented in the yearbooks are based on fertility reports of individual nations, there is a possibility that the criteria used to define fertility measures may vary among different nations. Therefore, researchers should scrutinize the data with caution. In this manuscript, I analyze male and female fertility data from the 2001 *Demographic Yearbook* which shows male and female fertility rates during the 1990–1998 period. Male and female TFRs in 43 countries and places during this time frame are examined cross-sectionally. Detailed findings will be shown in Chapter 4 of this book.

3.1.2 The Demographic and Health Surveys (DHS)

In recent years, fertility surveys that incorporate men have also taken place in some less developed countries. Among them, the Demographic and Health Surveys (DHS) is one of the important international surveys that include males in their questionnaires. Demographic and Health Surveys (DHS) are nationally-representative household surveys that provide data for a wide range of monitoring and impact evaluation indicators in the areas of population, health, and nutrition in developing countries (http://www.measuredhs.com/aboutsurveys/dhs/start.cfm). Initiated by the U.S. Agency for International Development (USAID), the DHS project is the third consecutive worldwide research project. Over the past 20 years, the DHS have been researching on topics of fertility, family planning, and mortality in many less developed nations. Since one of the key focuses of the DHS is to enhance the use of *household* health facility information by policy makers and program managers, household members, including *husbands* have been included in a number of the DHS surveys. By 2005, the DHS have conducted surveys of males or husbands in 42 countries, particularly in sub-Saharan Africa (Demographic and Health Surveys, 2005). Survey data that are released by the DHS present valuable male fertility information for developing countries. Now the DHS is considered as a leader in the field of demographic and health research on both men's and women's fertility and reproductive heath in developing countries.

3.1.3 The World Fertility Surveys (WFS)

The WFS is another international survey that collects fertility data of men. As one of the most important international undertakings in demographic data collection and analysis, the WFS and the Contraceptive Prevalence Surveys (CPS) are two predecessors of the DHS. The WFS focuses on investigating women's complete marriage and pregnancy histories, their socioeconomic background, contraception, breastfeeding, and fertility preferences. Three levels of information is collected by the WFS program. First is the community level. Second is the household level, which collects information on the age, sex, marital status, family relationships of all members of the household, and lifetime and current fertility. The third level information is the individual respondent selected for detailed interview. Over 40 developed and less developed countries have participated in the WFS project (Sprehe, 1974). Since fertility information of *household members* is gathered by the WFS surveys, fertility data for men are available for a few countries (Greene & Biddlecom, 2000). As the WFS has considerable scientific interest in providing comparable data on fertility for populations whose socioeconomic characteristics differ widely, fertility data released by the WFS may also be used to study factors affecting men's fertility from a comparative and international scope.

3.1.4 The National Survey of Family Growth (NSFG) Cycle 6

Besides the above data sources, several census or survey data have been carried out by individual nations presenting male fertility information. In the United States, for example, the 2002 National Survey of Family Growth (NSFG), Cycle 6, for the first time includes men in its surveys. The NSFG Cycle 6 was conducted by National Center for Health Statistics (NCHS), with the participation and funding support of nine other programs of the U.S. Department of Health and Human Services (http://www.cdc.gov/nchs/about_nsfg.htm). According to the NCHS, the NSFG Cycle 6 collects information on "family life, marriage and divorce, pregnancy, infertility, use of contraception, and men's and women's health" in the United States (National Center for Health Statistics, 2004, p. 5). The survey results are used by the U.S. Department of Health and Human Services and others to plan health services and health education programs. The survey results and data are also released to public and researchers to conduct studies of families, fertility, health and related issues.

In terms of the sample design, Cycle 6 was based on an area probability sample, which represents the household population of the U.S., 15–45 years of age. The survey sample was designed to produce national data rather than estimates of individual states. Following a voluntary and confidential rule, 7,643 women and 4,928 men were interviewed on topics of "fertility, marriage, cohabitation, contraception and related issues" (National Center for Health Statistics, 2005, p. 5).

The most important indicator of male fertility in Cycle 6 is number of biological children born to the male respondents. Demographers often refer this measure to children ever born (CEB). The equivalent measure of female fertility is based on the question that asks the female respondents' children ever born. Since Cycle 6 also presents the male and female respondent's demographic and socioeconomic characteristics along with information on a wide range of covariates, I use this dataset to conduct individual level analyses examining male and female fertility determinants. Research results are shown in Chapter 6 through 9.

3.1.5 Other U.S. Surveys Containing Male Fertility Information

In addition to the 2002 NSFG Cycle 6 dataset, several other U.S. surveys have also incorporated male fertility information in their questionnaires. Those surveys include: the Current Population Survey (CPS) conducted by the Bureau of Census, the Panel Study of Income Dynamics (PSID) funded by the National Science Foundation, the Survey of Income and Program Participation (SIPP) conducted by the U.S. Census Bureau, the National Survey of Families and Households (NSFH) carried out by the National Center for Health Statistics, the National Longitudinal Survey of Youth (NLSY) conveyed by the Bureau of Labor Statistics, and the National Survey of Adolescent Males (NSAM) (Thomas, 1996). These survey data provide valuable sources to study fertility of men in the United States.

3.2 Taiwan-Fukien Demographic Fact Book

Beyond the data sources discussed above, there is also an international data source that present information on male fertility in Taiwan. The Ministry of the Interior of Republic of China has published a series of *Taiwan-Fukien Demographic Fact Book*. This book presents birth data of Taiwan by mothers and by fathers from 1949 to the present (The Ministry of the Interior of Republic of China, 2005). This is a relatively complete national dataset that presents longitudinal male fertility rates of a single nation. Part of the macrolevel analysis of this book that will be shown in Chapter 5 is based on investigating this particular dataset.

3.3 The Quality of Male Fertility Data

I have discussed the readily available male fertility data sources, including those to be analyzed in this book. I now turn to discussion of an important issue that is usually associated with statistical analysis of male fertility, that is, the quality of male fertility data. This issue is important because underreporting of births occurs more often by men than by women, which is especially the case among younger age groups and in unions outside of marriage (Poston & Chang, 2005). In earlier chapters, I have pointed out that women are usually assumed to be more trustworthy than men when it comes to fertility because they are more directly involved in reproductive events such as pregnancies and births. For some fertility parameters such as miscarriages, fecundity-impairing illnesses and age of children, information provided by females are also claimed to be more reliable than reports given by males (Yaukey, Roberts, & Griffith, 1965). These factors have raised the concern of the quality of male fertility data. In the following subsections of the chapter, I endeavor to address this issue by reviewing previous literature that deals with this topic, which also helps me to justify the quality of some data to be analyzed in this book.

Regarding the quality and reliability of men's reports on fertility and fertility-related issues, previous demographic and sociological research has shown inconsistent results. Some studies suggest that men tend to underreport considerably the number of children born to them, especially children outside of marriage and from previous marriages. In a study assessing the retrospective fertility histories of men, Rendall and associates find that among the U.S. and British samples, one third to half of men have underreported their nonmarital births and births in previous marriages (Rendall, Clarke, Peters, Ranjit, & Verropoulou, 1999). Other studies show similar results. For instance, using the 1979 and 1980 Current Population Survey (CPS), Cherlin and colleagues (1983) indicate that children from previous unions living elsewhere are substantially missed in the reports of men when these reports are compared to those of women. Studies analyzing the 1987 wave of the National Survey of Families and Households (NSFH) also show large shortfalls in men's reports. Researchers reveal that between one quarter and one half of the children of nonresident fathers have been omitted by male respondents in the NSFH (J. A. Seltzer & Brandreth, 1994; Sorensen, 1997). Analyzing male data from the Survey of Income and Program Participation (SIPP) conducted in 1992 by the U.S. Census Bureau, Bachu (1996) finds higher nonresponse rates for men than for women, especially among the never-married population. She therefore suggests that "analysis of fertility data for single men requires much caution" (Bachu, 1996, p. 31). Rendall and associates (2006) assess men's fertility reports in the 2002 National Survey of Family Growth (NSFG) and show that men tend to underreport the number of their biological children. They contend that this is especially the case among men in younger age groups. Studies in Europe also note that women report family events with greater accuracy than men do (Auriat, 1991; Courgeau, 1992; Poulain, Rianey, & Firdion, 1992). Other fertility measures, such as infancy deaths, are found more likely to be omitted by males than by their female counterparts as well (W. Seltzer, 1973).

Although the above studies suggest the inaccuracy of male fertility data, other research exhibits that data gathered from men in certain social contexts are reliable and information on some fertility-related items reported by men is even more accurate than that collected from women. Zarate's (1967) study of the Latin American samples shows that Latin American males can provide sufficient information on CEB. Fikree, Gray, and Shah (1993) compare the reports of reproductive histories of spouses in a U.S. community and find that even though men's reporting of spontaneous or induced abortion is less reliable, their reports of timing and number of live births are accurate. Bachu (1996) evaluates the quality of data gathered from men in the SIPP and affirms the overall validity of men's responses, particularly the responses of married men. She states, "overall, extremely close agreement was found in the average number of CEB reported by all husbands (2,249 births per 1,000) and wives (2,248 births per 1,000)"(Bachu, 1996, p. 20). For the married population, Bachu (1996, p. 14) notes that "asking about the number of children they had ever fathered will yield the analyst with not much more information than if a survey was taken with the traditional 'female only' universe." By analyzing data from the NSFH, Bachrach and associates (1992) reach a similar conclusion. In addition, the results of a telephone survey conducted by Coughlin, LaPorte, O'Leary and Lee (1998) also reveal that men appear to be able to recall reproductive information (such as contraceptive use, frequency of intercourse and time of spouse's conception) with acceptable accuracy, and that American men's reports can be valid sources for epidemiological studies. These statements certify the accuracy of fertility reports by men.

Beyond the above analyses, a few other studies focusing on African populations further confirm the validity of reports by men. Hertrich (1998) has designed a field survey in a village of Mali to evaluate the quality of men's and women's responses to marital history among 78 marriages and reproductive history among 72 couples. The results show that women are not necessarily the best source of information on pregnancies. Researchers find that women are more likely to underreport pregnancies as compared to their husbands' reports, even though infancy death is more likely to be omitted by men. In another area that is related to fertility, marriage history, it is revealed that men can actually provide more reliable and detailed information than women because they are more directly involved in handling weddings and other related matters. In another study, Ratcliffe, Hill, Harrington and Walraven (2002) have surveyed 1,315 men and 1,261 women in rural Gambia. They report that even in Gambia where polygyny and marital disruption yield complicated reproductive histories for both men and women, men can report their wives' pregnancy events reliably. Interestingly, the authors observe that "women's refusals and reluctance to participate were more common than men's. . .the women were less willing to give details about children who had died and more easily upset by the recollection of dead children" (Ratcliffe et al., 2002, p. 582). These findings emphasize the value and importance of surveying men when it comes to fertility and fertility-related behaviors.

Given the mixed findings shown in previous studies, how to evaluate the discrepancies on male fertility reports shown in prior research becomes an important subject to consider. Several reasons may have resulted in the inconsistent results exhibited in prior studies. First, how the proper reference group is chosen affects the justification of the reliability of male responses. A major approach used by prior studies to justify the accuracy of the reports by men is to match the reports of men to those of women. This approach can be problematic because women's answers are not always true, which has been pointed out by previous studies (Hertrich, 1998; Jones & Forrest, 1992). Thus, the reference groups that have been relied on in previous studies can be a cause of incongruity occurred in previous analyses. Some researchers therefore recommend referring to some other sources of information besides women's announcements to justify the reliability of male fertility data. Ratcliffe and associates (2002), for example, compare both men's and women's reports to the records of demographic surveillance systems in local Gambia to judge the accuracy of male data. Future research may depend on other available sources such as regional vital registrations to evaluate male reports.

The second reason regards the variation of sample data applied in various studies. Discrepancies of previous analyses may lie in the fact that the samples were chosen from a variety of societies, which makes it difficult to draw a general conclusion regarding overall data accuracy. As Ratcliffe and colleagues (2002) indicate, men can provide reliable information about pregnancy events that their wives have experienced in rural Gambia, but "such complete knowledge may not be the case in other populations . . . especially where pregnancies outside of marriage are common" (Ratcliffe et al., 2002, p. 584). Due to sample variation, the results of studies may vary among different populations. The impression given by previous studies is that fertility information reported by married men is accurate in most societies. The sample variation among diverse subpopulations may challenge this presumed accuracy, which requires researchers to evaluate the comparability of male samples before drawing a general conclusion.

The last reason pertains to the representative ability of male samples. In other words, whether the male samples can accurately represent the male population being studied influences the consistency of previous studies. This reason is somehow related to the second reason discussed above. In a study of the Gambian population, Ratcliffe and associates (2002) show difficulties interviewing men due to their greater mobility as compared to women. Among such a population, without applying possible strategies to ensure that each men in the population has an equal possibility of being selected, then male samples chosen by the study are likely to be overrepresented by men who are less likely to migrate than others. Such a sampling approach may bias the conclusions because men who are less mobile may have different reproductive attitudes and behaviors as compared to those who migrate more frequently. In this sense, discrepancies may occur due to sampling strategies applied in the analyses. That is why researchers contend that complete knowledge of men on some fertility events found in a population may not be applied to other groups (Ratcliffe et al., 2002). These findings remind researchers to address the issue of sample representative ability to alleviate incongruities among previous studies.

Despite mixed findings regarding the accuracy of male fertility reports, prior studies reflect the fact that men can be a valuable source providing reliable fertility information in some populations. This finding makes it plausible to rely on men's biographies that describe their fertility history, their own characteristics and socioeconomic status to estimate male fertility variation. The use of first hand male fertility data avoids the biases that may be generated by merely relying on women's reports of their partners' characteristics. As Zarate (1967) indicates, "[although] women may be in a better position to provide accurate information on several aspects of childbearing, it is doubtful that they are in a position to provide better information on [men's] socioeconomic factors" (Zarate, 1967, p. 849). Men's detailed reporting on some fertility related items, such as marital history, supplements the shortfalls of women's reports.

As far as the quality of male fertility data to be analyzed in this book, the problem of underreporting births by men in the NSFG dataset has indeed been pointed out by Rendall and associates (Rendall et al., 2006). They assess fatherhood at ages 18–27 years old in the period of 1991–2000. The reason they choose this group of male respondents is because data problems are normally greatest at younger ages. Their evaluation results show that underreporting of fatherhood for this group of men does exist in the NSFG dataset, meaning applying this dataset to examine male fertility outcomes could be problematic. Considering this matter, when I use the NSFG data to examine male fertility, I break the analysis into two parts for comparison purposes. Part one excludes males under 25 years of age and part two has all male respondents included. Put differently, I compare results with and without younger men to justify whether including younger men who has a greater possibility of underreporting births significantly changes the research results. Doing so also helps to assess the quality of male fertility data presented by the NSFG Cycle 6. Applying age 25 to differentiate the male samples is based on the median age at first marriage of 26 for the U.S. men in year 2003 reported by the U.S. Census Bureau. The criterion of age at first marriage is used because prior research suggests that unmarried younger men have a higher likelihood of underreporting births than other men (Poston & Chang, 2005). I now move to statistical methods to be employed in this book.

3.4 Statistical Methods

3.4.1 *Descriptive Analysis and Ordinary Least Square (OLS) Regression*

Basic descriptive methods are used throughout the empirical analysis of this book. Within Chapters 4 and 5, I present basic descriptive tables of data that show male and female fertility rates and ratios. Such descriptive analysis helps to show male and female fertility trends and patterns, and particularly the male and female fertility differentials in rates. The descriptive tables in the following chapters (Chapters 6, 7, 8, and 9) that analyze the individual level data demonstrate, for most covariates, the percentage distributions of cases. For continuously measured variables, such as age, the mean values are shown in descriptive tables. All of the descriptive tabulations are weighted based on sample weights given by the NSFG. The sample weights will be discussed in a more detailed manner in paragraphs introducing survey commands by using Stata in the following sub-sections.

The ordinary least square (OLS) regression is used in Chapter 5 when examining male and female fertility in Taiwan. The dependent variables in the chapter are male and female TFRs. The independent variables are a number of covariates that are drawn from theoretical explanations of female fertility changes in Taiwan.

3.4.2 *The Poisson Regression Models*

The microlevel statistical models in Chapters 6, 7, 8, and 9 are Poisson regression models. The Poisson regression model is considered as the appropriate statistical procedure to be used because the dependent variable at the microlevel, CEB, is a count variable. When examining count variables, the Poisson model is superior to ordinary least squares (OLS) or other linear models because the distribution of a count variable, such as CEB, is one that is heavily skewed with a long right tail, especially in the cases of low fertility populations. The skewed distribution of the CEB could be due to the observed distribution of data having a very low mean, which reflects many women desiring few children and few women wanting many children in low fertility countries. Poisson regression is the suitable procedure to estimate CEB also because CEB is a positive integer. OLS is appropriate only if the dependent variable, the count, is independently and identically distributed. Since the CEB distribution does not meet such an assumption, applying the linear regression model to CEB in this case could result in "inefficient, inconsistent, and biased estimates" (Long & Freese, 2006). Thus, the Poisson regression model is applied in this research, which can be expressed as follows:

$$\mu_i = \exp(a + X_{1i}b_1 + X_{2i}b_2 + \cdots + X_{ki}b_k + \varepsilon_i)$$

Where μ_i is the expected number of counts for the ith observation, which is estimated from observed characteristics of the independent variables; b_i represents deviation from the mean of the omitted category, which is the reference group. The X variables are related to μ nonlinearly. In this case, μ_i is the expected number of children born to a respondent based on the respondent's demographic and socioeconomic characteristics and so forth. All cases are weighted by using Stata survey commands based on the final weights of each sample given by the NSFG.

When interpreting the Poisson regression results, I exponentiate the b coefficients to odds ratios which Stata refers to as incidence rate ratios (IRR). Throughout this monograph, odds ratios about 1 indicate a higher likelihood of having children for a particular category of the independent variable. Those below 1 signify a reduced likelihood of giving births to children. The percentage change in odds ratios is another way to show the effects of covariates. A positive percentage change in odds ratios indicate a positive influence of a covariate on the dependent variable (CEB); and a negative value of percentage change in odds ratios displays a suppressing effect of a covariate on CEB.

In the Poisson regression models, I also incorporate the gender interaction terms to evaluate whether the effect of a particular variable on the dependent variable (CEB) varies by gender. In other words, the gender interaction term allows examining whether a particular variable has significantly different effects on men's and women's CEBs. This strategy is commonplace in the social science literature, which in this research allows for a statistical testing of fertility differentials by gender within the multivariate context. The interaction effect exists if an X variable's effect does depend on the values of other X variables (Allison, 1999). In this case, if the gender interaction effect exists, then an X variable's effect on CEB depends on the values of the gender variable, that is, whether the gender variable is coded as "male" or "female."

The most common approach for modeling interaction is to introduce cross-product terms of the explanatory variables into the multiple regression models. In the analysis, I first combine the male and female respondent data files together. I then generate a gender variable, which is coded as "1" if the respondent is a male and "0" if otherwise. The gender interaction terms (or cross-products) are created by multiplying the gender variable and each covariate I am interested in examining. If the gender interaction terms (or cross-products) are statistically significant at the 0.05 level, then I claim the effect of a particular covariate on the dependent variable varies by gender. Put differently, significant differentials exist between male and female fertility outcomes due to the effect of a particular independent variable. In this research, I define the reference group as females. Positive regression coefficients (or odds ratios above 1) suggest a stronger effect of a particular variable on male fertility than on female fertility.

3.4.3 Sample Weights and Survey Commands Using Stata

In complex survey designs, such as the NSFG survey design, samples are often stratified by variables of interest to ensure a balanced number of respondents for each category of the variable. For example, in regions with an unbalanced distribution of racial and ethnic groups, the stratification strategy may be used to ensure that a particular racial or ethnic group is not over- or under-represented by survey samples. Besides stratification, survey samples are usually clustered in complex survey designs as well. In the case of NSFG Cycle 6, both stratification and clustering strategies are applied. For instance, in the NSFG surveys, households were sampled first, and then the respondents were chosen from sampled households. Such stratification and clustering approaches, however, can skew the standard errors from statistical analyses. Because significance levels are affected by standard errors, the conclusions drawn from a statistical model that does not consider the stratification and clustering issues may not be accurate. To adjust the standard errors to correct for those complex survey design factors, Stata survey commands are employed in the regression models, which takes sample weights into account.

The Stata survey command is expressed as "svyset" followed by "pweight," "strata" and "psu." Such a command is used to specify the stratification scheme, sampling weights and primary sampling units in the NSFG data. The keyword "strata" specifies the stratification variable, in the case of Cycle 6, is "sest." "Pweight" and "psu" specify the weight variable and primary sampling unit, respectively. The NSFG user's guide indicates that "final poststratified and fully adjusted weight [is] (FINALWGT)," which "is located in columns 4873–4890 in the Female Respondent file, . . ., and columns 2927–2944 in the Male file" (National Center for Health Statistics, 2004, p. 9). Thus, "pweight" should be "finalweight" in the NSFG Cycle 6 datasets. "Psu" is "secu," according to the user's guide. All these keywords are combined in a single command line, which is expressed as:

Svyset [pweight = finalweight], strata (sest) psu (secu)

This expression should be placed before running any descriptive analysis or regression models. For the descriptive analysis, for example, the "svymean" command is placed before the name of a continuous variable to yield the mean value for such a variable; and the "svydes" command is set before the name of the categorical variable so that the percentage distribution of the case can be presented in a Stata output. As to the Poisson regression models, the command "svy:" should be added before the Poisson regression commands. Taking these complex sample features into account will permit replication of the nationally representative estimates that appear in published NCHS reports. The discussion of survey commands by Stata used in the analysis also allows researchers to replicate results presented in this manuscript.

3.5 Summary

This chapter introduces a number of available male fertility data sources, including those to be examined in this book. The chapter also discusses and evaluates the quality of male fertility reports. Discrepancies are found regarding the reliability of data collected from men. Such discrepancies are considered to be caused by the manner in which the reference group is chosen, different sampling strategies, and the variation of sample data among diverse populations. Despite the discrepancies shown in previous research, I argue that fertility data gathered from men can still be valid data sources among certain populations. Reliable male fertility data have strong merits in terms of learning male fertility trends and its determinants. The Poisson regression modeling, with coefficients interpreted in the form of odds ratios, is the prime statistical methodology. The microlevel analysis chapters will rely mainly on Poisson regression method and employ a consistent format, which facilitates concordance between chapters and eases interpretation throughout the analysis. Chapter 4 and other following individual chapters will detail the datasets, the methodology and specific measures used.

References

Allison, P. (1999). *Multiple regression*. Thousand Oaks, CA: Pine Forge Press.

Auriat, N. (1991). Who forgets? An analysis of memory effects in a retrospective survey on migration history. *European Journal of Population, 7*(4), 311–342.

Bachrach, C. A., Evans, V. J., Ellison, S. A., & Stolley, K. S. (1992). *What price do we pay for single sex fertility surveys?* Paper presented at the Population Association of America (PAA) Annual Meeting, Denver, Colorado.

Bachu, A. (1996). *Fertility of American men*: U.S. Census Bureau Population Division Working Paper, No.14.

Cherlin, A., Griffith, J., & McCarthy, J. (1983). A note on maritally-disrupted men's reports of child support in the June 1980 current population survey. *Demography, 20*(3), 385–389.

Coleman, D. A. (2000). Male fertility trends in industrial countries: Theories in search of some evidence. In C. Bledsoe, J. I. Guyer, & S. Lerner (Eds.), *Fertility and male life-cycle in the era of fertility decline* (pp. 29–60). New York: Oxford University Press.

Coughlin, M. T., LaPorte, R. E., O'Leary, L., & Lee, P. A. (1998). How accurate is male recall of reproductive information? *American Journal of Epidemiology, 148*(8), 806–809.

Courgeau, D. (1992). Impact of response errors on event history analysis. *Population: An English Selection, 4*, 97–110.

Fikree, F. F., Gray, R. H., & Shah, F. (1993). Can men be trusted? A comparison of pregnancy histories reported by husbands and wives. *American Journal of Epidemiology, 138*(4), 237–242.

Greene, M. E., & Biddlecom, A. E. (2000). Absent and problematic men: Demographic accounts of male reproductive roles. *Population and Development Review, 26*(1), 81–115.

Hertrich, V. (1998). Are men's and women's answers to be equally trusted? A dual collection of birth and marriage histories in a population in Mali. *Population: An English Selection, 10*(2), 303–318.

Jones, E. F., & Forrest, J. D. (1992). Underreporting of abortion in surveys of U.S. women. *Demography, 29*(1), 113–126.

Long, J. S., & Freese, J. (2006). *Regression models for categorical dependent variables using stata* (2nd Edn). College Station: Stata Press.

National Center for Health Statistics (2004). *Public use data file documentation, national survey of family growth cycle 6: 2002, user's guide*. Hyattsville, MD, National Center for Health Statistics.

National Center for Health Statistics (2005). *Fertility, family planning and reproductive health of U.S. women: Data from the 2002 national survey of family growth*. Hyattsville, MD: National Center for Health Statistics.

Poston, D. L. J., & Chang, C.-F. (2005). Bringing males in: A critical demographic plea for incorporating males in methodological and theoretical analyses of human fertility. *Critical Demography, 1*(1), 1–15.

Poulain, M., Rianey, B., & Firdion, J.-M. (1992). Data from a life history survey and the Belgian population register: A comparison. *Population: An English Selection*, *4*, 77–96.

Ratcliffe, A. A., Hill, A. G., Harrington, D. P., & Walraven, G. (2002). Reporting of fertility events by men and women in rural Gambia. *Demography*, *39*(3), 573–586.

Rendall, M. S., Clarke, L., Peters, H. E., Ranjit, N., & Verropoulou, G. (1999). Incomplete reporting of men's fertility in the United States and Britain: A research note. *Demography*, *36*(1), 135–144.

Rendall, M. S., Joyner, K., Peters, H. E., Yang, F., Handcock, M. S., & Ryan, A. (2006). *A Bayesian approach to combining population and survey data for male fertility estimation*. Paper presented at the annual meetings of population association of America, Los Angeles, California.

Seltzer, W. (1973). *Demographic data collection: A summary of experience*. New York: The Population Council.

Seltzer, J. A., & Brandreth, Y. (1994). What fathers say about involvement with children after separation. *Journal of Family Issues*, *15*(1), 49–77.

Sorensen, E. (1997). A national profile of nonresident fathers and their ability to pay child support. *Journal of Marriage and the Family*, *59*(4), 785–797.

Sprehe, J. T. (1974). The world fertility survey: An international program of fertility research. *Studies in Family Planning*, *5*(2), 35–41.

The Ministry of the Interior of Republic of China (2005). *Taiwan-Fukien demographic fact book*. Taipei, Taiwan: Ministry of the Interior of Republic of China.

Thomas, V. S. (1996). *The age pattern of male fertility in the U.S. 1957–1964 birth cohorts* Unpublished Dissertation. Duke University, Durham, NC.

United Nations (2001). *Demographic yearbook 2001*. New York: United Nations.

Yaukey, D., Roberts, B. J., & Griffith, W. (1965). Husbands' vs. wives' responses to a fertility survey. *Population Studies*, *XIX*(1), 29–43.

Zarate, A. O. (1967). A note on the accuracy of male responses to questions on fertility. *Demography*, *4*(2), 846–849.

Part II
Male and Female Fertility Differentials in Rates

Chapter 4
A Cross-Sectional Analysis of Male and Female Fertility in 43 Countries and Places, 1990–1998

Fertility levels have long been key components of population changes (Bongaarts & Bulatao, 2000). They are important elements to study because the level of fertility determines the population age and sex structure and, in turn, leads to a wide range of social and economic changes. For instance, fertility levels alter cohort sizes, which impact a full set of age-graded institutions such as the social security system, schools, the labor force, and marriage. In recent decades, fertility levels have shown a dramatic decline. Such a decline is referred to the fertility transitions which is composed by three stages: relatively high and stable fertility, followed by a period of fertility decline, and then followed by relatively low and stable fertility (Morgan & Hagewen, 2005). The fertility transitions are observed to have completed in many developed countries and are in progress in much of the rest of the world. The demographic transition theory that is based on the fertility transition model has been formed to explain fertility changes associated with social and economic transitions (Notestein, 1953).

The fertility transition model, however, is built primarily according to the changing levels of female fertility. Whether male fertility has experienced similar transitions has not been fully explored in previous literature. Moreover, the demographic transition theory has been mainly performed to account for female fertility declines. Whether the demographic transition theory and other demographic theories of fertility need to be revised, extended or elaborated when they are applied to male fertility remain unquestioned. In order to address these issues, I analyze male fertility levels through comparing them to those of females in Chapter 4 and 5 of this manuscript. Additionally, I apply demographic theories based on female fertility to model male fertility changes in Chapter 5. By combining both cross-sectional and longitudinal perspectives in these chapters, I show in detail how male fertility differs from female fertility in rates cross-sectionally in Chapter 4 and longitudinally in Chapter 5. The research evidence of these two chapters suggests that male fertility levels cannot be fully represented and explained by fertility levels of females. Further, I show that existing demographic theories do not account for male fertility as well as they explain female fertility at the aggregate level. In this research, fertility levels for both sexes are measured by fertility rates, specifically, the total fertility rate (TFR) and the age-specific fertility rate (ASFR).

L. Zhang, *Male Fertility Patterns and Determinants*, The Springer Series on Demographic Methods and Population Analysis 27, DOI 10.1007/978-90-481-8939-7_4,

This chapter will start with a brief review of prior literature on comparative studies of male and female fertility. It then moves to the analysis of male and female total fertility rates (TFRs) during 1990–1998 in 43 countries and places, followed by an analysis of male and female age-specific fertility rates (ASFRs) in these regions. Finally, I conclude findings and discuss implications of this research.

4.1 Research Background

As discussed in Chapter 2, comparing male and female fertility differentials is a major topic covered by previous studies of male fertility. In general, researchers find that male fertility cannot be fully represented by female fertility. When using completed measures of fertility, such as the net reproduction rate (NRR) and the total fertility rate (TFR), to represent fertility, male and female fertility rates are found to be non-identical (Coleman, 2000; Kuczynski, 1932). In most developed regions studied, the general pattern shown in previous research is that male fertility was first higher than female fertility and the reverse pattern became true in later years (Ventura, Martin, Curtin, Matthews, & Park, 2000; Zhang, Poston, Dudley, & Chang, 2007).

With regard to age-specific fertility, researchers demonstrate very different male and female fertility patterns resulted from the effect of age. Male fertility is found to have a later and lower peak, and remaining higher than that of female's with increasing age (1994). Men are also observed to start having their first births later as compared to women. Moreover, the first birth distribution of men is found to be more dispersed than that of women in many populations (Coleman, 2000; Thomas, 1996).

This current research attempts to extend the above literature in the following aspects: First, previous studies examining male and female completed fertility levels have focused primarily on more developed countries which have male fertility data readily available. Thus far, male fertility patterns and rates in less developed nations with higher fertility rates have hardly been studied. In this research, I employ data from the United Nations *Demographic Yearbook* to extend the analysis to some high fertility countries that have been underrepresented in previous studies. Second, most prior literature reveals male fertility change from a longitudinal point of view. Researchers show how male and female fertility differ over time. This study takes a cross-sectional perspective instead to demonstrate the manner in which male fertility differs from female fertility during a specific time frame. By doing so, I am able to link the male and female fertility differentials to the level of total fertility at the aggregate level.

As to the studies of age-specific fertility, though Paget and Timaeus's (1994) research is especially informative in exploring men's age-specific fertility patterns as compared to those of women, there is still room to improve their research. For instance, Paget and Timaeus's (1994) results are based on examining male and female fertility during 1959–1980 when fertility rates were generally high. Such comparison results may need to be updated after a dramatic fertility decline has taken place in most countries in recent decades. Additionally, Paget and Timaeus's

(1994) study examines male fertility of a mixed group of countries with various fertility levels. Those countries include four polygynous populations, eight high fertility populations, and five medium fertility populations. It will be interesting to group countries and places into low and high fertility countries and to show male and female fertility differ. The analysis in the following sub-sections will fill these gaps of prior research.

4.2 Data

As discussed in previous chapters, many studies have been undertaken during the past on modeling and describing female fertility. In contrast to the attention paid to female fertility, little work has been done analyzing male fertility. Part of the reason for this downplay of men in fertility is that data on male fertility are relatively difficult to obtain. Both birth registration data and surveys are usually tabulated according to the age of mothers rather than fathers. It is "particularly difficult to locate data of an acceptable quality, especially for high-fertility countries" (Paget & Timaeus, 1994, p. 335). In recent years, some data sources that contain male fertility information have become available, which provides researchers the opportunity to study male fertility. The United Nations *Demographic Yearbook* is one of those major data sources that present male fertility information. It compiles birth data for both sexes in several of its special editions. Fertility data presented in the *Demographic Yearbook* are gathered by sending out a set of questionnaires by the United Nations annually and monthly to national statistical services and other appropriate government offices in world countries. The United Nations explain that "data forwarded on these questionnaires are supplemented, to the extent possible, by data taken from official national publications and by correspondence with the national statistical services" (United Nations, 2001, Genral Remarks, p. 3).

This research uses data presented in the *Demographic Yearbook 2001-Special Topic: Natality Statistics.* This data source provides information on live-birth rates specific for age of mother and father from 1990 to 1998. The age-specific fertility rates (ASFRs) presented in Tables 7 and 9 in the 2001 *Demographic Yearbook* are generated by relying on the reports of live births by age of mother and father during 1990–1998 shown in Tables 6 and 8 in the same data source. The numerator for calculating the ASFR is the number of births by mothers or by fathers that are presented in Tables 6 and 8; and the denominator is the number of females or males in the population for a particular age group. I rely on the ASFRs presented in the 2001 *Demographic Yearbook* to investigate male and female fertility trends and patterns in this chapter. Totally, 43 (out of 229) countries and places are included in this research. These regions are chosen because they have both male and female fertility data available, which serves the purpose of analyzing fertility from gendered and comparative perspectives. For countries and places with more than one year of fertility data available during the 1990–1998 period, male and female fertility rates that represent the most recent year are chosen. Fertility data analyzed in this chapter are based on records of all births, both legitimate and illegitimate.

4.3 Measures

Male fertility in this research is operationalized into two fertility measures, which are the total fertility rate (TFR) and the age-specific fertility rate (ASFR). The same measures are applied to female fertility. The TFR represents the total number of live births a hypothetical (synthetic) cohort of 1,000 men or women would end up having if they passed through their reproductive years and if they were subjected to the ASFRs of a specific region in a particular year. The calculation of the TFR for females is well-known, namely, the summing of a schedule of the ASFRs, and then multiplying of the sum by five, the width of the age interval of the ASFRs. For females, seven ASFRs (15–19, 20–24, . . . 40–44, 45–49) are used in the calculation. That is:

$$\text{TFR} = \sum_{x=15}^{49} ASFR$$

In this study, births to mothers under age 15 or over 50 are included in the ASFRs for 15–19 and 45–49, respectively. Male TFRs are calculated in the same way, but because both male fecundity and fertility extend beyond age 49, nine ASFRs (15–19, 20–24, . . . 50–54, 55–59) are employed. Births to fathers under age 15 or over 60 are included in the ASFRs for 15–19 and 55–59, respectively.

The following formula depicts the way the ASFR for females is calculated:

$$ASFR_{women,\ age\ x\ to\ x+n} = \left(\frac{births_{women,\ age\ x\ to\ x+n}}{midyear\ population_{women,\ age\ x\ to\ x+n}}\right)^{*} 1,000$$

The male ASFRs should be calculated in the same way, but the numerator changes to number of births given by males in a certain age group and the denominator changes to number of male population in a certain age group. The ASFRs analyzed in this chapter come directly from the *2001 Demographic Yearbook-Special Topic*.

4.4 Results

4.4.1 Male and Female TFRs

Table 4.1 presents the names of the 43 countries and places, along with their corresponding male and female TFRs during 1990–1998, and the specific years chosen for the analysis. Among the 43 countries and places studied, females have a mean TFR value across the 43 countries and places of 1,958 with a standard deviation of 723.5. Female TFRs vary from a high of 3,914 in Mexico to a low of 871.5 in Hong Kong. Males have an average TFR value among the 43 countries and places of 2,008 with a standard deviation of 889.4. The highest male TFR is 4,705 in Mexico and the lowest is 867.5 in Hong Kong.

Table 4.1 Male and female TFRs in 43 selected countries and places, 1990–1998

Country	Abbreviation	Male TFR	Female TFR	Selected year
Australia	AUS	1835.5	1855.0	94
Bahamas	BAH	2277.0	1954.0	92
Bahrain	BRN	1953.5	2783.0	97
Bosnia and Herzegovina	BIH	1624.0	1744.5	91
Bulgaria	BUL	1064.5	1093.0	97
Canada	CAN	1458.0	1551.5	97
Chile	CHI	2163.5	2146.5	98
China-Hong Kong	HKG	867.5	871.5	98
China-Macao	MAC	1311.5	1037.0	98
Croatia	CRO	1605.5	1683.0	97
Cuba	CUB	1409.5	1439.5	96
Cyprus	CYP	1839.5	1918.5	98
Denmark	DEN	1672.0	1759.0	96
Egypt	EGY	4205.5	3742.5	95
El Salvador	ESA	3692.5	2937.5	98
Estonia	EST	1184.0	1240.0	97
Greenland	GRN	1755.0	2369.0	98
Hungary	HUN	1318.5	1335.0	98
Iceland	ISL	2015.5	2040.0	97
Israel	ISR	3154.0	2933.0	97
Italy	ITA	1202.0	1191.5	95
Kyrgyzstan	KGZ	3023.5	2827.0	98
Latvia	LAT	1055.5	1111.0	97
Lithuania	LTU	1302.5	1363.5	98
Mauritius	MRI	2027.0	2036.0	97
Mexico	MEX	4705.0	3913.5	90
Norway	NOR	1855.5	1923.0	91
Panama	PAN	3173.0	2910.5	97
Philippines	PHI	3708.0	3259.0	91
Poland	POL	1490.5	1507.0	97
Portugal	POR	1507.0	1465.0	97
Puerto Rico	PUR	2071.0	1913.0	98
Romania	ROM	1349.0	1332.0	98
Singapore	SIN	1645.0	1706.5	97
Slovenia	SLO	1061.0	1233.5	98
Spain	ESP	1191.5	1186.0	97
The former Yugoslav Rep. of Macedonia	MKD	1896.0	1926.5	97
Trinidad and Tobago	TRI	1809.0	1718.0	97
Tunisia	TUN	3111.0	2614.0	95
United States	USA	1914.5	2032.5	97
Uruguay	URU	2332.0	2464.5	96
Venezuela	VEN	2812.5	2248.0	96
Yugoslavia	YUG	1843.0	1896.0	95

Note: The female TFR for Australia is based on the reports of the U.S. Census Bureau International Data Sheet to adjust the very high female TFR reported in the *Demographic Yearbook*.
Source: The United Nations *Demographic Yearbook* 2001, Tables 7 and 9.

The average male TFR in the 43 countries and places is only slightly higher than the average female TFR by a difference of 49 births per 1,000 persons. The two countries and places with the highest, and the lowest, TFR values for females and males are the same, namely, Mexico and Hong Kong. Male TFRs do show more variation than female TFRs, as evidenced by their respective standard deviations and coefficients of relative variation (CRV) of 0.44 and 0.37 (CRV is the standard deviation divided by the mean). The more variation of male TFRs indicates a larger variance in male fertility than in female fertility in human societies, which echoes findings of previous research.

I then correlate the male and female TFRs and get a value of 0.96, which is very high and statistically significant. Such a finding suggests that at the country level, male and female fertility levels represented by the TFRs tend to be more similar than dissimilar among countries examined. Then does the high correlation mean that male fertility can be replaced by female fertility? The analysis in the following sub-sections provides answers to this question.

Figure 4.1 presents a scatterplot of male and female TFRs for these 43 countries and places, using the data in Table 4.1. The countries and places in this figure are identified by abbreviated versions of their names (see Table 4.1 for the abbreviations). The unity line inside the figure is not a regression line, which indicates that geographic areas above this unity line have higher female than male TFRs with the opposite for countries and places below the line. The general pattern shown by Fig. 4.1 seems to be consistent with the descriptive results discussed earlier. That is, male and female TFRs in most locales studied are comparable, considering that most of the countries and places are either close to or fall on the unity line.

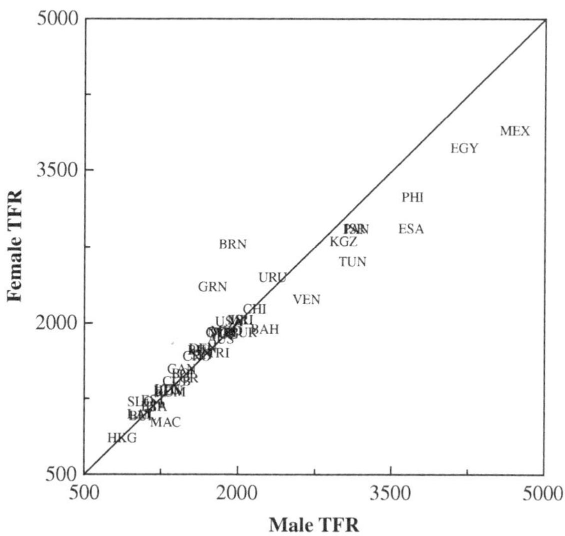

Fig. 4.1 Male and Female TFRs: 43 Countries and Places: 1990–1998
Source: The United Nations *Demographic Yearbook* 2001, Tables 7 and 9.

One important observation drawn from Fig. 4.1, but not shown by the descriptive analysis, however, is that male and female TFRs are closer in values in countries and places that have both male and female TFRs lower than 2,200. In those countries and places, female fertility tends to be higher than male fertility, considering most of those countries and places are above the unity line. For countries and places that have male and female TFR values above 2,200, they tend to have dissimilar male and female TFRs since they are relatively more far away from the unity line. Meanwhile, countries and places that have male and female TFR values above 2,200 are scattered below the unity line, suggesting that in high fertility countries and places, male fertility tends to be higher than female fertility (see Fig. 4.1).

Based on the above findings, important implications may be drawn: First, the male and female fertility differentials are more likely to exist in high fertility (TFR > 2,200) than in low fertility (TFR < 2,200) countries. In those high fertility countries and places, male fertility tends to be higher than female fertility. Second, low fertility countries tend to have comparable male and female fertility. However, in those low fertility countries and places, there is still a fertility gap by gender with female fertility slightly higher than male fertility. According to these implications, the high correlation between male and female fertility shown in the earlier analysis is possibly due to the fact that the majority of the countries and places studied are low fertility regions.

Besides the TFRs, the ratio of male to female TFRs (R_{TFRs}) is also used to mea sure the relationship between male and female fertility. The calculation of R_{TFR} follows the following formula:

$$R_{TFR} = \frac{MaleTFR}{FemaleTFR}$$

Here a R_{TFR} value of 1.0 represents identical male and female TFRs. A R_{TFR} value above 1.0 means that male TFR is higher than female TFR, with the opposite for a R_{TFR} value below 1.0. Results based on examining the R_{TFR} values are consistent with findings drawn from Fig. 4.1. That is, the majority of the R_{TFRs} values in 43 countries and places are found to be lower than 1.0, meaning that female TFRs are higher than male TFRs in most countries and places. Those countries and places have male and female TFRs lower than 2,200.

To further demonstrate the dissimilar, rather than similar, patterns of male and female total fertility in high fertility countries and places (TFRs > 2,200), Fig. 4.2 plots the residuals from a regression equation with the values of male TFRs that are predicted by female TFRs. In this figure, countries and places below the line have predicted values of male fertility larger than their actual values, with the opposite for countries and places above the line.

Figure 4.2 suggests that knowledge of female fertility predicts male fertility well for most countries and places. It does especially well for countries and places with low male and female TFRs (TFRs < 2,200), such as Canada (CAN), Australia (AUS) and Singapore (SIN). In these regions, errors predicting male TFRs with female TFRs are small. With the predicted male TFRs above 2,200, the errors increase dramatically. For instance, Tunisia (TUN) has an actual male TFR of 3,111, but a

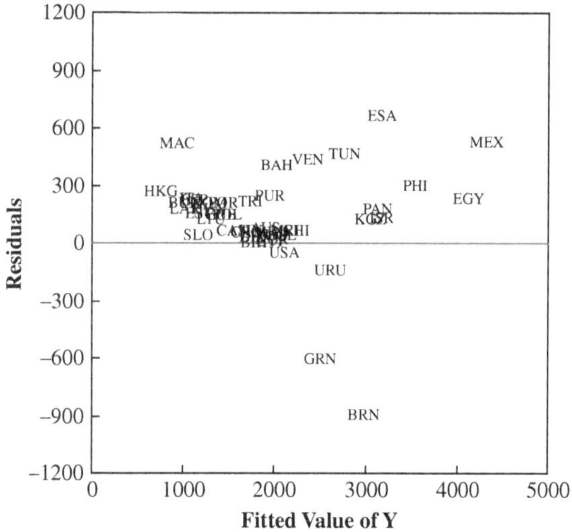

Fig. 4.2 Residuals vs. Fitted Y Values: 43 Countries and Places: 1990–1998
Source: The United Nations *Demographic Yearbook* 2001, Tables 7 and 9.

predicted value of 2,779, an under-prediction of 332 births. Venezuela (VEN) has an actual male TFR of 2,654, but a predicted value of 2,348, an under-prediction of 306 births. At the other extremes, Bahrain (BRN) has an actual male TFR of 1,953, but a predicted male TFR of 2,978, or an over-prediction of 1,025 births. Greenland (GRN) has an actual male TFR of 1,755, but a predicted value of 2,491, for an over-prediction of 736 births; El Salvador (ESA) has an actual male TFR of 3,692, but a predicted value of 3,196, for an under-prediction of 497 births. These findings again confirm that male fertility is different from female fertility, especially in high fertility regions.

To summarize findings of the above analysis, male and female fertility show similar rates in lower fertility countries, with female fertility slightly higher than male fertility. The male and female differences in TFRs mainly occur in high fertility (TFRs > 2,200) regions where male fertility is higher than female fertility. Therefore, a TFR value of 2,200 or *replacement level fertility* for the study period of 1990–1998 seems to be a critical value distinguishing male and female fertility patterns at the aggregate level. This is the most important finding of this chapter. I will discuss the significance of this finding in a greater detail in the conclusion part. Since the TFR is generated from the ASFRs, the next section of this chapter moves to the analysis of age-specific fertility, delving more into how age effects shape the male and female fertility relationships.

4.4.2 Male and Female ASFRs

Paget and Timaeus's (1994) have used the Gompertz model to show effectively the age-specific patterns of male and female fertility. They have described male fertility as starting later, having a lower peak and stopping much later as compared

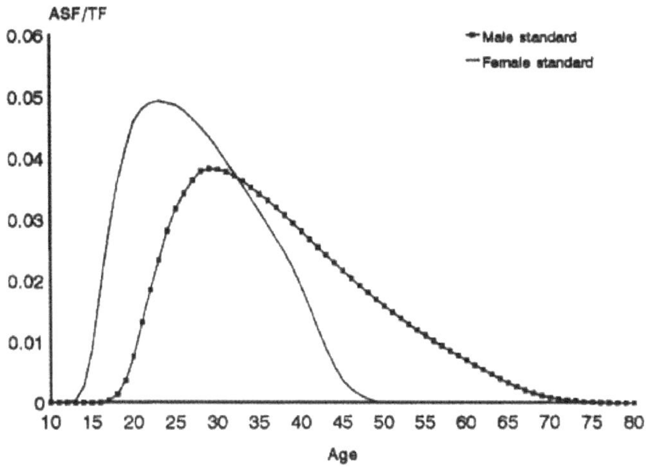

Fig. 4.3 Male and female standard fertility distribution
Source: Fig. 1 in Paget and Timaeus's (1994) study, p. 337.

to female fertility. Such a pattern is demonstrated in Fig. 4.3 which was constructed by Paget and Timaeus (1994). In this study, I rely on contrasting the mean values and the ratios of male and female ASFRs to carry on Paget and Timaeu's study. Since I am interested in contrasting the male and female age-specific fertility differentials in high and low fertility countries, I also break down the 43 countries and places into high and low fertility regions according to the critical TFR value of 2,200. Countries with male and female TFRs higher than 2,200 are classified as high fertility countries and countries with male and female TFRs lower than 2,200 are considered as low fertility countries. Among the 43 countries and places, nine of them have both male and female TFR values above 2,200. They are considered as high fertility countries and the rest, 34 of them, are defined as low fertility regions. Thus, in contrast to Paget and Timaeus's samples which are composed primarily by countries with high and medium levels of fertility, samples in this research to a large extent represent low fertility locales.

For the purpose of comparing male and female fertility rates, the ASFRs for seven age groups (15–19, 20–24, . . . 40–44, 45–49) are examined in this part of the study. Tables 4.2 and 4.3 show the descriptive analysis of male and female ASFRs for the seven age groups in high and low fertility countries, respectively. According to the mean values of male and female ASFRs presented in column 1, it is clear that female fertility rates surpass those of males for younger age groups (15–19, 20–24, and 25–29). It is especially the case for the youngest age group, 15–19. The average value of female ASFRs for this age group is about five times that of males in both high and low fertility countries. The fertility gap between males and females decreases as age increases. Staring from age group 30–34, the opposite situation is true, that is, the average value of male ASFRs begins to be larger than that of females. For instance, the average ASFR for age group 30–34 is 167.9 for men and 127.3 for women in high fertility countries; and the corresponding values are

89.6 and 71.8 in low fertility countries. In fact, the gap between the mean values of male and female ASFRs tends to increase after age 34. Male ASFRs continue to be higher than female ASFRs until later age groups. For age group 45–49, in particular, the mean value of male ASFR in high fertility countries is 37.9, which is almost six times the average female ASFR. In low fertility countries, the ratio of average male to female ASFR is even higher (around ten) for the same age group. After age 49, female fertility stops while male fertility continues to later ages. These findings are generally consistent with results shown in Paget and Timaeus's (1994) research on age-specific patterns of male fertility. Some new findings also emerge in this research, which will be elaborated in the following paragraphs.

I next transform the information presented in Tables 4.2 and 4.3 to Fig. 4.4 which graphs the mean values of the ASFRs for different age groups for both males and females in high and low fertility regions. As it can be seen, age group 30–34 seems to be the threshold at which male fertility begins to be higher than female fertility for both high and low fertility countries (see Fig. 4.4). Female ASFRs are higher than male ASFRs before a population approaches this age group; and

Table 4.2 Descriptive analyses of male and female ASFRs in high fertility countries, 1990–1998 ($N=9$)

	Mean		Std. Dev.		Min.		Max.	
	Male	Female	Male	Female	Male	Female	Male	Female
15–19	14.7	60.5	13.4	40.5	0.0	13.4	32.5	105.7
20–24	85.9	147.3	52.4	34.2	6.0	91.2	169.9	210.8
25–29	154.2	167.9	39.7	41.6	90.5	128.5	229.7	250
30–34	167.9	127.3	42.5	30.3	114	92.1	242.6	176.6
35–39	125.3	75.4	38.5	19.9	76.4	53.9	196.5	107.6
40–44	73.5	25.8	22.8	9.1	41	15.1	108.9	40.5
45–49	37.9	6.5	14.4	4.3	16.3	1.2	57.6	14.3

Source: See Table 4.1.

Table 4.3 Descriptive analyses of male and female ASFRs in low fertility countries, 1990–1998 ($N=34$)

	Mean		Std. Dev.		Min.		Max.	
	Male	Female	Male	Female	Male	Female	Male	Female
15–19	5.7	29.1	5.9	18.1	0.4	5.3	29	73.8
20–24	48.3	89.4	24.3	33.1	10.8	25	99.8	161.5
25–29	93.3	100.7	30.1	23.4	31.7	56.5	188.5	140.3
30–34	89.6	71.8	26.2	25.4	42.3	22.4	156.9	133.2
35–39	52.4	31.7	18.9	17.9	18	7.3	92.1	104.4
40–44	22.4	7.1	12.2	7.4	6.4	1.6	68.0	45.9
45–49	8.6	0.8	8.6	1.9	2.0	0.1	51.7	10.9

Source: See Table 4.1.

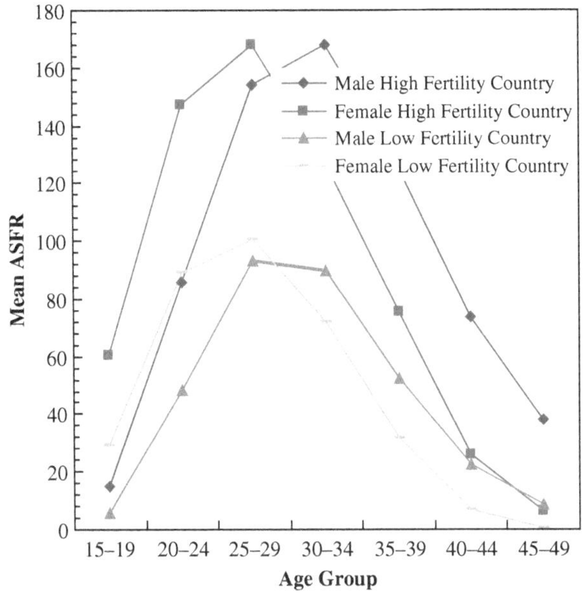

Fig. 4.4 Mean Values of Male and Female ASFRs for High and Low Fertility Countries, 1990–1998
Source: The United Nations *Demographic Yearbook* 2001, Tables 7 and 9.

the opposite situation is true once a population reaches this age group regardless the level of total fertility. Such findings fall in line with the age-specific fertility patterns for both sexes shown in Paget and Timaeus' (1994) research that is presented in Fig. 4.3. The consistency suggests that the threshold effect of age group 30–34 on differentiating male and female age-specific fertility is independent of the variation of total fertility. This is a new finding that adds to the existing literature.

Regarding the standard deviations of male and female ASFRs, the general pattern shown in Tables 4.2 and 4.3 emphasizes that for younger age groups (15–19 and 20–24), female ASFRs tend to vary to a larger extent than those of males. The reverse pattern appears to be the case for the rest of the older age groups. These results imply that at the aggregate level, the general statement that there is a greater variation among male fertility than among female fertility may not be true when fertility of younger age groups is considered. The general statement is perhaps valid when total fertility is taken into consideration. This is a finding that has not been shown in prior studies.

Table 4.4 presents the descriptive analysis of the ratios of male and female ASFRs (R_{ASFRs}), which are calculated based on the following formula:

$$R_{TFR} = \frac{MaleASFR}{FemaleASFR}$$

Table 4.4 Descriptive analyses of ratios of male and female ASFRs, 1990–1998 (N1 = 9 for high fertility countries and N2 = 34 for low fertility countries)

	Mean		Std. Dev.		Min		Max	
	H	L	H	L	H	L	H	L
15–19	0.18	0.19	0.11	0.10	0.00	0.04	0.33	0.45
20–24	0.54	0.53	0.27	0.17	0.07	0.19	0.82	0.88
25–29	0.93	0.94	0.20	0.27	0.61	0.43	1.15	1.75
30–34	1.32	1.32	0.08	0.37	1.23	0.56	1.48	2.64
35–39	1.65	1.82	0.17	0.50	1.40	0.73	1.83	3.63
40–44	2.93	3.65	0.52	1.21	1.96	1.48	3.74	7.46
45–49	8.17	24.19	4.15	15.72	2.11	2.00	15.25	86.00

Note: "H" indicates high fertility countries and "L" indicates low fertility countries.
Source: See Table 4.1.

Results in Table 4.4 show that the mean values of the R_{ASFRs} for high and low fertility regions are similar before a population reaches the age group of 40–44. Afterwards, the mean values of R_{ASFRs} in low fertility countries are significantly higher than those in high fertility countries. For age group 45–49, in particular, the mean value of the R_{ASFR} is 24.2 in low fertility countries and 8.2 in high fertility countries. One may argue that the much higher mean value of R_{ASFR} in low fertility nations for this age group may be caused by a larger standard deviation of the R_{ASFRs}, which is influenced by the number of observed cases.

To justify this argument, Figs. 4.5 and 4.6 show the R_{ASFRs} for seven age groups in high and low fertility regions, respectively. Apparently, the majority of the R_{ASFRs} for age group 45–49 in low fertility regions range from 15 to 40; whereas the values of the R_{ASFRs} in high fertility regions are between 2.1 and 15.3. This means that the R_{ASFR} for age group 45–49 in countries with TFR values below 2,200 is indeed higher than that in countries with TFRs above 2,200. Such a difference is not likely to be caused by their non-identical standard deviations. These results, coupled with findings drawn from Tables 4.2 and 4.3, suggest that the fertility differentials by sex in older age groups increase with total fertility decreases. In this sense, the reduction of total fertility rate does affect the male and female fertility correlation.

4.5 Conclusion and Discussion

In this chapter, I have explored male fertility through comparing fertility rates of men to those of women. Several important findings are obtained from this research. First, in terms of total fertility, I find that male and female TFRs are not identical at the country level. They tend to be similar in countries and places with TFR values lower than 2,200 where female fertility is slightly higher than male fertility. In countries and places with both male and female TFRs above 2,200, male and female fertility are likely to be more dissimilar than similar; and male fertility is higher than female fertility. I therefore claim that *replacement-level fertility* can be an indicator

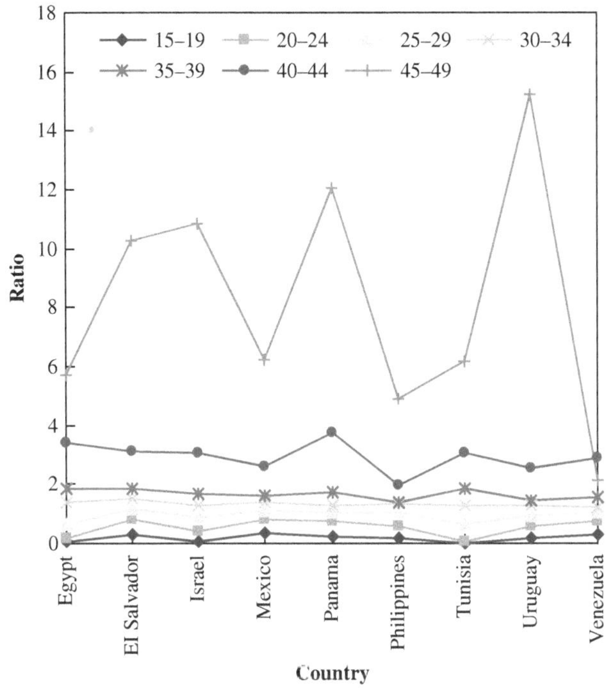

Fig. 4.5 Ratios of male and female ASFRs: high fertility countries, 1990–1998
Source: The United Nations *Demographic Yearbook* 2001, Tables 7 and 9.

describing the correlation of male and female total fertility rates. This is an important finding because previous research has been emphasizing various time points that shape the total fertility gap by sex. Prior studies show a general pattern of male fertility being higher than female fertility in earlier years and the opposite relationship became the case afterwards. Those studies, however, are not able to explain why the time points when male and female fertility had crossovers vary by region (Coleman, 2000; Poston & Chang, 2005; Ventura, Martin, Curtin, Matthews, & Park, 2000). In European countries, the male and female TFR crossovers occurred in the 1950s–1960s; whereas in the United States and in Taiwan, the crossover years occurred almost 40 years later. Coleman (2000) argues that the shortage of men associated with two world wars should be a cause of the changing relationship of male and female fertility. This argument is not a feasible explanation for the case of non-European regions.

The finding of *replacement-level fertility* being an indicator of the male and female fertility correlation shown in this research probably provides a better justification to the above phenomenon. The rationale behind the finding is that it is replacement-level fertility rather than the time effect that shapes the fertility differentials by sex. Once total fertility reaches to the replacement level, male and female fertility crossover occurs and female fertility begins to be higher than male fertility. Such a conclusion may not be attained from studies taking a longitudinal point of view.

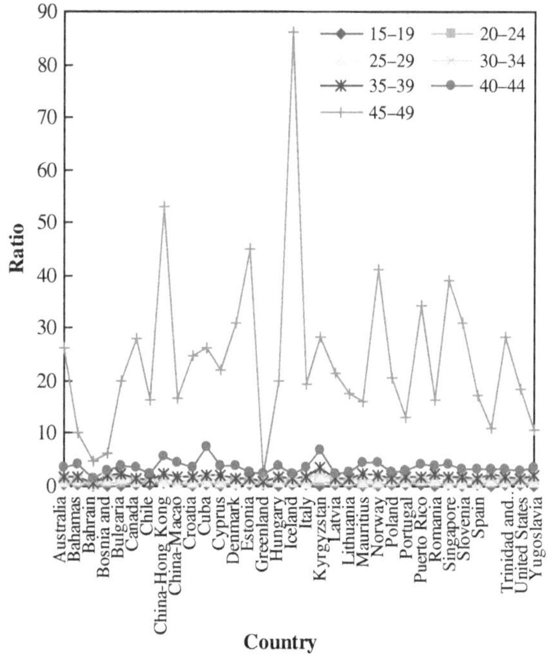

Fig. 4.6 Ratios of male and female ASFRs: low fertility countries, 1990–1998
Source: The United Nations *Demographic Yearbook* 2001, Tables 7 and 9.

Then why does replacement-level fertility differentiate the male and female fertility patterns? Another question to ask is that why male fertility was first higher than female fertility and then it declined to a lower rate after the TFR drops below the replacement level. Here I propose several possible explanations to address these questions. First, immigration and emigration may interact with the level of fertility in determining the male and female fertility association. Countries and places with fertility levels higher than the replacement level are likely to be more developed countries. These countries and places tend to have higher immigration than emigration rates. Since migration is usually dominated by younger males, more developed countries are thus likely to have more men than women in their populations due to immigration, especially in younger age groups. As a result, the denominator for calculating male fertility is larger for more developed countries than for less developed countries. If the male fertility rate is calculated by using the number of births given by females in the same age group as the proxy of births given by males, then the relatively larger denominator for males will lead to a lower male than female fertility rate. The opposite situation applies to less developed countries with TFRs higher than the replacement level. This explanation elucidates why replacement-level fertility determines the male and female differentials in TFRs.

The second explanation links the level of fertility to mortality differentials by sex. As we know, females generally enjoy a longer life expectancy and a lower mortality than males. Though the sex differentials in mortality are universal, the mortality gap by sex varies across regions and over time. In more developed countries, better socioeconomic conditions, more advanced social welfare system and health care may shrink the mortality gap by sex. If this is the case, then relatively more men are eliminated from the denominator of the fertility equation in less developed countries. As a result, male fertility is higher than female fertility in those countries where total fertility is above the replacement level.

Finally, I propose that cultural preferences of some societies may explain the differentials of male and female fertility. In Taiwan, for example, there is a strong cultural preference for a male heir. Thus, the sex ratio at birth (SRB) in this particular locale has been severely out of balance, particularly in recent years when fertility declines to a below replacement level. One of the consequences of the unbalanced SRB is that a large number of surplus men emerge in the marriage market simply because there are not enough brides for them to marry (Poston & Zhang, 2007). Considering this situation, I hypothesize that the relatively lower availability of females in the marriage market in recent years may have led to a higher percentage of females being married than males. Since the majority of births in Taiwan occur in marital unions, a higher marital rate of females may have resulted in a higher female than male fertility. All these explanations are proposed hypotheses, which will need to be tested and verified by empirical analysis in future.

Besides focusing on studying male and female TFRs, this chapter has also presented several findings regarding the age-specific fertility differentials by sex. The age effects shown on male and female fertility fall in line with results presented in Paget and Timaeus' (1994) analysis. In addition, the study presents some findings that have not been elaborated in previous literature: (1) The age group of 30–34 is revealed in this study to be the threshold defining the male and female age-specific fertility differentials. Female fertility has a higher rate than male fertility before a population reaches this age group. Afterwards, males begin to have higher fertility than females, especially in age groups 40–44 and 45–49. These results, coupled with Paget and Timaeus' (1994) findings, suggest that the threshold effect of age group 30–34 does not seem to vary over time with the changing level of total fertility. Put differently, the threshold effect of age group 30–34 on differentiating male and female fertility is immune from the reduction of total fertility rate. (2) A higher male than female fertility in older age groups is especially apparent in low fertility countries (TFR < 2,200). This finding suggests that in this sense, the male and female age-specific fertility differentials interact with the level of total fertility. This interaction effect may be caused by the age and sex structure of a population. This is because lower fertility countries are usually featured by relatively more mature population structures. Consequently, there is a higher percentage of older females than males in those populations. Thus, the denominator for calculating male fertility in low fertility countries becomes smaller than that for females. The male age-specific fertility in older age groups, in turn, becomes higher in low fertility countries than in higher fertility countries. Such fertility differentials by sex in older age groups are therefore more apparent in low fertility than in high fertility countries. This finding implies that older age groups in low fertility countries may become the target population of future research that is interested in exploring fertility differentials in rates by sex.

According to the above summarized findings, I make some projections on future male fertility trends and patterns. Future male fertility at the aggregate level in most countries will be in a similar declining pattern as female fertility. Under the low fertility regime, the total fertility differentials by sex will shrink with female fertility being slightly higher than male fertility. When age specific fertility is taken into consideration, the fertility gap by sex will persist regardless the reduction of total fertility. Since the male and female age specific fertility differentials are shown mainly in very young ages and age groups above 45, incorporating male fertility into fertility studies may be far more important in countries with young or mature population structures.

Thus far, I have examined male and female fertility rates and showed that male fertility levels cannot be fully represented by those of females. The chapter, however, has not spoken to another important demographic issue, that is, whether demographic theories based on female fertility variation can be applied to male fertility. The next chapter that studies male and female fertility in Taiwan and the following chapters that analyze male and female fertility in the United States will concentrate on exploring this theme.

References

Bongaarts, J., & Bulatao, R. A. (2000). *Beyond six billion: Forecasting the world's population*. Washington, DC: NAS Press.

Coleman, D. A. (2000). Male fertility trends in industrial countries: Theories in search of some evidence. In C. Bledsoe, J. I.Guyers, & S. Lerner (Eds.). *Fertility and male life-cycle in the era of fertility decline* (pp. 29–60). New York: Oxford University Press.

Kuczynski, R. R. (1932). *Fertility and reproduction*. New York: Falcon Press.

Morgan, S. P., & Hagewen, K. J. (2005). Fertility. In D. L. J. Poston, M. Micklin (Eds.), *Handbook of population* (pp. 229–251). New York: Springer.

Nations, U. (2001). *Demographic yearbook 2001*. New York: United Nations.

Notestein, F. W. (1953). Economic problems of population change. *Proceedings of the eighth international conference of agricultural Economists*. New York: Oxford University Press.

Paget, W. J., & Timaeus, I. M. (1994). A relational gompertz model of male fertility: Development and assessment. *Population Studies, 48*(2), 333–340.

Poston, D. L. J., & Chang, C.-F. (2005). Bringing males in: A critical demographic plea for incorporating males in methodological and theoretical analyses of human fertility. *Critical Demography, 1*(1), 1–15.

Poston, D. L. J., & Zhang, L. (2007). How many extra boys have been born in China? In X. Zheng, D. L. J. Poston, & B. Gu (Eds.), *Gender and sexually transmitted infections in China*. Beijing: Beijing University Press.

Thomas, V. S. (1996). *The age pattern of male fertility in the U.S. 1957–1964 birth cohorts*, Unpublished dissertation. Durham, NC: Duke University.

Ventura, S. J., Martin, J. A., Curtin, S. C., Matthews, T. J., & Park, M. M. (2000). *Births: Final Data for 1998*: National Vital Statistics Reports 48.

Zhang, L., Poston, J., Dudley, L., & Chang, C.-F. (2007). Male and female fertility in Taiwan. In J. Poston, L. Dudley, & W. Yang (Eds.), *The family and social change in Chinese societies*. New York: Springer.

Chapter 5
Male and Female Fertility in Taiwan: Trends and Transitions, 1975–2004

The previous chapter has examined the total fertility and the age-specific fertility patterns for males as compared to those of females cross-sectionally among countries. This chapter investigates male fertility in a specific region, namely, Taiwan, from both longitudinal and cross-sectional points of view. The locale of Taiwan is chosen because it has detailed male fertility data readily available. Studying male fertility in Taiwan also has a significant meaning because Taiwan represents one of those regions that have experienced substantial fertility declines and have completed the demographic transition. Prior research has documented a dramatic fertility decline of Taiwanese females from about 6.5 children per woman in the mid-1950s to fewer than two children per woman in the mid-1980s (Poston 2000). Today, fertility of Taiwanese women is far below the replacement level and Taiwan is considered as one of the lowest-low fertility regions in the world. However, the picture of fertility transition in Taiwan is not complete until the dynamics of male fertility is brought into the research scope. This research aims to fulfill the picture by exploring male fertility trends and transitions in this specific location. Results shown in this analysis may also be generalized to other regions that have experienced similar fertility reduction.

5.1 Study Objectives

This chapter has three objectives. The first is to investigate the trends and transitions of male and female fertility in Taiwan. I show how male fertility differs from female fertility measured in TFRs and ASFRs. Second, I intend to explore how male and female fertility rates are impacted by social and economic factors at the aggregate level. Since *Taiwan-Fukien Demographic Fact Book*, one of the major data sources of this research, provides fertility data across age and educational groups, my analysis also examines how education plays a role in differentiating male and female fertility across age groups. Education in this research is classified into six categories according to *Taiwan-Fukien Demographic Fact Book*-illiterate, self-taught, primary graduated, junior graduated, senior graduated, and university or college graduated. The final objective of this research is

L. Zhang, *Male Fertility Patterns and Determinants*, The Springer Series on Demographic Methods and Population Analysis 27, DOI 10.1007/978-90-481-8939-7_5,

to address the demographic concern raised in Chapter 4 that is, whether fertility theories explaining demographic transitions of females can account for male fertility change. I use several major theories explaining female fertility transitions in Taiwan to predict male fertility changes in 23 sub-regions of Taiwan in 2002.

5.2 Data, Measures and Methods

Two primary sources of data are employed in this study: *Taiwan-Fukien Demographic Fact Book* and *National Statistics Reports*. The first data source is published by the Ministry of the Interior of Republic of China, which presents birth data of Taiwan by mothers and by fathers from 1949 to the present (Ministry of the Interior of Republic of China, 2005, p. 329). The book also presents male fertility rates in 23 sub-regions of Taiwan for a number of years. Thus far, it is one of the data sources that present the most complete fertility information of Taiwan. The second data source is released by the Statistics Bureau of the Republic of China. This data source contains statistics on population, industry, labor force, social security and a number of other important indicators. The statistical reports are available since the 1960s to the most recent year. These two data sources have provided researchers tremendous opportunities to explore fertility transitions in Taiwan. As Collver and associates describe, "since 1961, detailed, reliable data have been published for all 361 minor administrative division of the [Taiwan] island, making it possible to record and analyze in detail an historic change of fertility at the moment when it is happening" (Collver, Speare, & Liu, 1967, p. 329).

In this research, I draw fertility data from 1976–2002 *Taiwan-Fukien Demographic Fact Book* and 2004 *National Statistics Reports*. I also rely on data from 1998 *National Statistics Reports* to represent variables measuring the socioeconomic condition and people's educational achievements in Taiwan. These socioeconomic and educational variables are used as the independent variables to predict fertility changes in 23 sub-regions of Taiwan. Since the dependent variables, male and female TFRs, is measured with data for year 2002, it is theoretically appropriate to posit temporally the independent variables five or so years before the onset of the dependent variable. Thus, data for year 1997 or 1998 are chosen in the analysis to represent values of the independent variables.

In terms of the measures, the TFR and the ASFR are used to operationalize male an female fertility. The measures used as independent variables that represent socioeconomic and educational status of Taiwanese in year 1997 or 1998 are: (1) percentage of males and females who were receiving or have received college degrees; (2) combined average family income; (3) infant mortality rate; (4) percentages of married males and females in age group 20–24; and (5) population density (per square kilometer). Descriptive analysis and the OLS regressions are major statistical methods applied in this research.

5.3 Results

5.3.1 Male and Female Fertility Trends and Transitions, 1975–2004

The first part of the analysis focuses on the trends and transitions of male and female fertility in Taiwan from 1975 to 2004. Given that different criteria have been used to generate fertility rates in *Taiwan-Fukien Demographic Fact Book* for years 1949–1974 and for years 1975 to present, I decided to focus only on years of 1975–2004 to avoid inconsistent results caused by data collection and compilation. Similar to Chapter 4 the calculation of female TFRs follows the following formula:

$$\text{TFR} = \sum_{x=15}^{49} ASFR$$

Where seven ASFRs (15–19, 20–24,... 40–44, 45–49) are used in the calculation for females. Since male fecundity and fertility extend beyond age 49, Ministry of the Interior of Taiwan applies nine ASFRs (15–19, 20–24,... 55–59) to yield male TFRs. When generating male and female TFRs, births to mothers under age 15 and over 50 are included in age groups 15–19 and 45–49, respectively. Births to fathers under age 15 and over 60 are included in age groups 15–19 and 55–59, respectively.

Figure 5.1 charts male and female TFRs for Taiwan for each year from 1975 to 2004. Both male and female TFRs have shown a dramatic declining pattern over time, especially during the 1970s to the mid 1980s. In 1975, the male and female TFRs were 3,255 and 2,765, respectively. The TFRs then dropped to 1,720 for males and 1,675 for females in year 1986. Until year 2004, both male and female TFRs were below the replacement level. Male TFR declined to 1,150 in 2004, which may be interpreted as follows: a hypothetical (synthetic) cohort of 1,000 men ended up having 1,150 live births, as they passed through their 45 years of fertility span and they were subjected to the ASFRs of Taiwanese men in 2004.

When male TFRs are compared to female TFRs, Fig. 5.1 shows that years 1975–1988 are the years that had higher male than female fertility rates. Since year 1989, female fertility rates have been higher than those of males. This differentiation can also be observed when examining the ratios (R_{TFR}) of male and female TFRs. The highest R_{TFR} occurred in 1975 with a value of 1.18, meaning that in 1975 male fertility was 18% higher than female fertility. In that year, there were 490 more births per 1,000 males than 1,000 females. The ratios then dropped year by year, approaching 1.0 in 1988 and below 1.0 afterwards. If we take a closer look at the TFR values for males and females in year 1998 when male and female fertility had a crossover, it may be noticed that both male and female TFRs were 1,885, which is about replacement-level fertility.

This is an interesting finding because it supports findings of the previous chapter that replacement-level fertility is the threshold defining the male and female fertility relationship. Male fertility is higher than that of females before fertility drops to

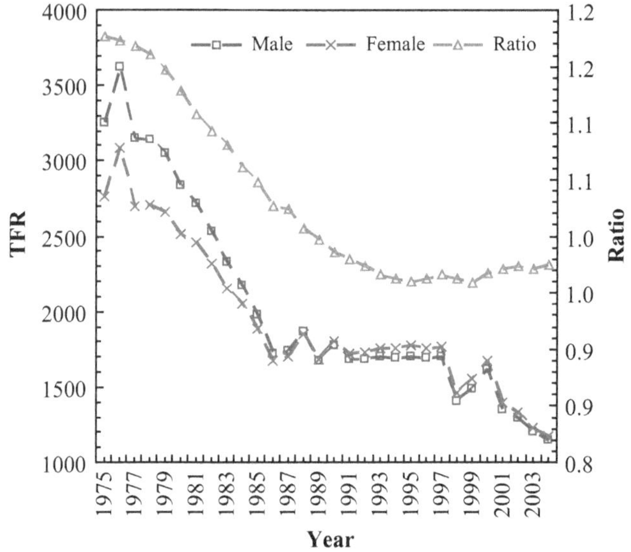

Fig. 5.1 Male and female TFRs and ratios of male and female TFRs: Taiwan, 1975–2004
Sources: Taiwan-Fukien *Demographic Yearbooks* 1976–2002 and *National Statistics Reports* 2004.

the replacement level; and the reverse pattern is true once the TFRs for both men and women are below the replacement level. In other words, the case of Taiwan confirms the validity of the general conclusion drawn from Chapter 4 Findings of this research also indicate that by the late 1980s, Taiwan had joined most of the developed world with female fertility being higher than male fertility. This important trend has largely gone unnoticed in the demographic literature because of the tendency of conventional demography to ignore males in fertility studies.

An additional point that needs to be made here regards the issue of handling unknown births in the dataset. Clarifying this issue may help the reader to better interpret the results. When compiling *Taiwan-Fukien Demographic Fact Book*. Ministry of the Interior of Republic of China has taken unknown births into consideration. Unknown births refer to those births whose fathers or mothers are not known or not reported. Two strategies have been used to handle unknown births when generating fertility rates in this data source. For years 1949–1974, unknown births are excluded from the calculation of fertility rates, such as the TFRs and the ASFRs, because ages of fathers or mothers for those unknown births cannot be identified. Since 1975, Ministry of the Interior of Republic of China indicates that "all births to fathers [or mothers] whose ages are unknown are proportionately distributed among those to fathers [or mothers] of known age in calculating age-specific fertility rates" (Ministry of the Interior of Republic of China, 2002, p. 22, 2005). Both strategies have limitations when dealing with unknown births because of the following reasons: First, the strategy of omitting unknown births for years 1949–1974 lowers the actual level of fertility because the numerators for calculating fertility rates become smaller. This is especially the case for males since men are more likely to underreport births than women, which is reflected by a higher percentage of unknown births by men than by women shown in Table 5.1. As it can be seen, in each year, a higher percentage of unknown births occurs to males than to females. The study in next section of male and female ASFRs will include years 1949–1974.

The strategy of proportionally distributing unknown births to various age groups for years 1975 to present also has a problem. This is because the strategy may bias the actual level of fertility in that not each age group has an equal probability of underreporting births. Unknown births are more likely to occur in younger age groups than in older age groups. For men, in particular, younger age groups may deserve to receive even higher percentages of unknown births than the actual proportions these groups have received in the dataset. So proportionally distributing unknown births to age groups would result in the ASFRs being smaller for younger

Table 5.1 Numbers of total births, unknown births and percent of unknown births for males and females: Taiwan, 1949–1974

		Male		Female	
Year	Total births	Unknown births	% Unknown births	Unknown births	% Unknown births
1949	300,843	7,991	2.66	420	0.14
1950	323,643	8,458	2.61	487	0.15
1951	385,383	10,971	2.85	712	0.18
1952	372,905	11,138	2.99	776	0.21
1953	374,536	10,750	2.87	945	0.25
1954	383,574	10,589	2.76	889	0.23
1955	403,683	11,034	2.73	1,058	0.26
1956	414,036	12,361	2.99	1,052	0.25
1957	394,870	9,930	2.51	1,031	0.26
1958	410,885	10,364	2.52	1,246	0.30
1959	421,458	10,022	2.38	1,258	0.30
1960	421,458	8,590	2.04	1,396	0.33
1961	419,442	7,647	1.82	1,548	0.37
1962	420,254	7,301	1.74	1,458	0.35
1963	423,469	5,445	1.29	42	0.01
1964	416,926	5,649	1.35	35	0.01
1965	406,604	5,336	1.31	60	0.01
1966	415,108	6,232	1.50	92	0.02
1967	374,282	4,820	1.29	105	0.03
1968	394,260	5,151	1.31	46	0.01
1969	390,728	4,973	1.27	86	0.02
1970	394,015	5,202	1.32	84	0.02
1971	380,424	4,817	1.27	86	0.02
1972	365,749	4,860	1.33	141	0.04
1973	366,942	4,894	1.33	120	0.03
1974	367,823	4,788	1.30	100	0.03

Source: Derived from *Taiwan-Fukien Demographic Fact Book* 1976. Table 13.

age groups whereas larger for older age groups than the actual fertility rates. Given that the percentages of unknown births to total number of births for men and women have been declining over time (see Table 5.1), fertility rates for the 1970s may be more accurate than those for earlier years. For years 1975 till present, considering that births in Taiwan mainly occur in marital unions, the strategy of proportionally distributing unknown births should not severely bias the actual fertility rates. From this perspective, I consider fertility data used in this research having a high accuracy, although readers should keep the issue of handling unknown births in mind when interpreting results of this chapter.

5.3.2 Male and Female ASFRs in Taiwan, 1949–2002

The next part of the analysis examines the age-specific fertility patterns for Taiwanese males and females from 1949 to 2002. I extend the study period back to year 1949 because the age-specific fertility patterns can be shown in a clearer manner over a longer period of time. In addition, since fertility is examined in separate age groups in this sub-section, the results should be less sensitive to biases due to applying different strategies collecting and compiling data as compared to TFRs. Figures 5.2 and 5.3 below show the ASFRs for males and females for each age group from 1949 to 2002, respectively.

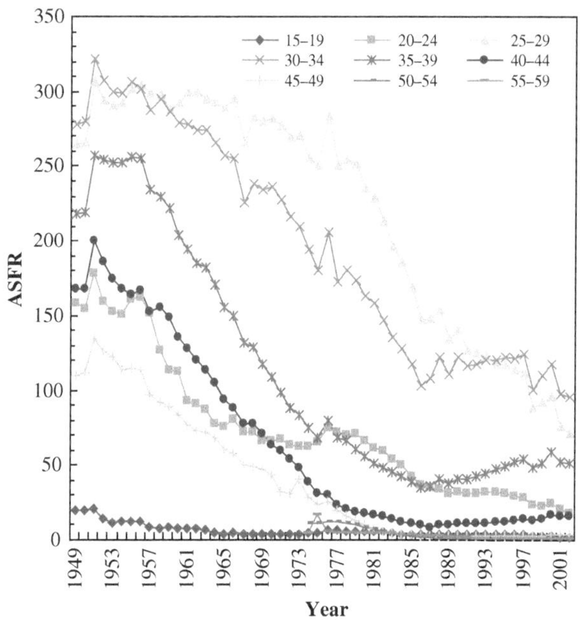

Fig. 5.2 Male ASFRs: Taiwan, 1949–2002
Sources: see sources for Fig. 5.1.

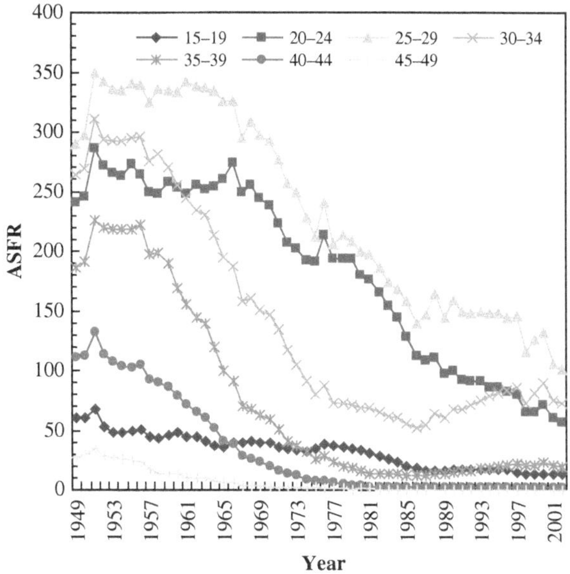

Fig. 5.3 Female ASFRs: Taiwan, 1949–2002
Sources: see sources for Fig. 5.1.

As it can be seen, both male and female ASFRs have been declining during the past 50 or so years. The fertility peaks for both sexes occur in age group 25–29 for most years. For this age group, the highest ASFR for males was 306 in year 1951 and the lowest ASFR was 71 in 2002, with a mean value of 221.3. For females, the corresponding values range from 350 in 1951 and 101 in 2002, with an average value of 235.2. Though males and females had their fertility peaks in the same age group for most years, females have shown a higher average value of ASFRs than males. Another observation drawn from Figs. 5.2 and 5.3 is that since the early 1990s, the male fertility peak has shifted to age group 30–34 though the fertility peak of women remains in age group 25–29. In this sense, the timing of having children for males is probably more sensitive than that for females due to modernization. Additionally, male fertility pattern is observed as starting later, stopping much later, and remaining higher in older ages than females. For males, for most years, the highest ASFRs occur in the age group 25–29, followed by age groups 30–34, 35–39, 20–24, 45–49, 50–54 and 55–59. For females, age group 25–29 has the highest ASFR values for most years, followed by age groups 20–24, 30–34, 35–39, 15–19 and 45–49. These differences again demonstrate the unique fertility pattern of males.

As far as the correlation of male and female ASFRs is concerned, the ratios of male and female ASFRs, R_{ASFRs}, are examined and presented in Fig. 5.4. It can be seen that the R_{ASFRs} are clustered according to age groups. The older the age group, the higher the R_{ASFRs} values. For instance, in year 1981, the male ASFR was seven times the female ASFR for the 40–44 age group. For age group 45–49, an even more dramatic fertility differential by sex is observed over time, with a maximum R_{ASFR} value of 28.0 in 1974. These findings again illustrate that male and female fertility

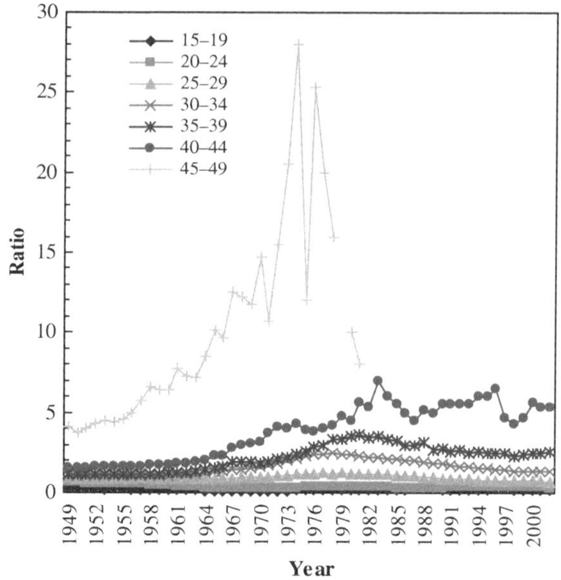

Fig. 5.4 Ratios of male and female ASFRs: Taiwan, 1949–2002
Sources: see sources for Fig. 5.1.

differentials by age mainly occur in older age groups, which is consistent to findings shown in Chapter 4. The trend line of R_{ASFRs} for age group 45–49 ends since the late 1970s because the female ASFRs became zero since then.

5.3.3 Male and Female Fertility Differentials by Educational Attainment, 1974–2002

I now extend the study of age-specific fertility by sex by incorporating educational attainments in the analysis. I examine the ratios of male and female ASFRs by level of education for seven age groups, which are shown in Figs. 5.5, 5.6, 5.7, 5.8, 5.9 and 5.10. Below I will describe fertility patterns revealed by each figure and then summarize findings and results.

Figure 5.5 demonstrates the ratios of male and female ASFRs by educational attainment for age group 15–19. For all educational groups, except for college or university graduates, the R_{ASFRs} are below 1.0. This makes sense because for younger age groups, females usually have a higher fertility than males. The R_{ASFRs} value for age group 15–19 stands out and is higher than 1.0, meaning that education plays a role in lowering female fertility to a greater extent than male fertility. The R_{ASFR} values are clustered based on educational attainments. In general, the higher the level of education, the higher the ratios of male to female ASFRs. This finding again suggests that a higher level of education is likely to reduce female fertility to a greater extent than male fertility. The trend line representing university or college

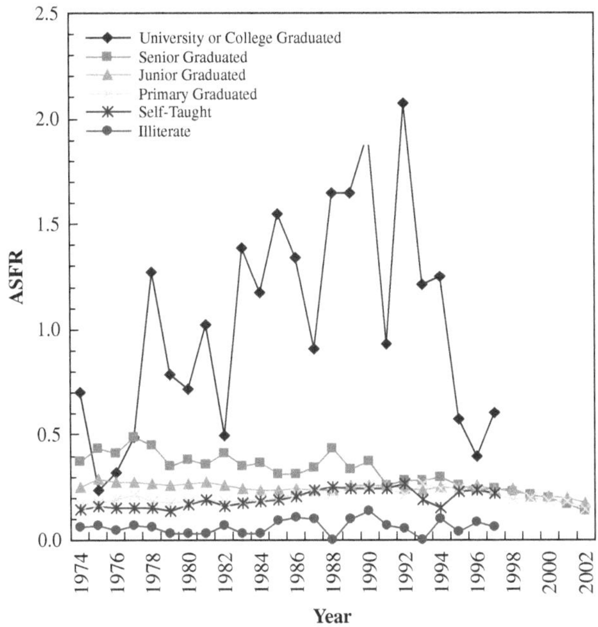

Fig. 5.5 Ratios of male and female ASFRs by educational attainment for age group 15–19: Taiwan, 1974–2002
Sources: see sources for Fig. 5.1.

graduates stops after 1997 because since then female ASFRs became zero. In general, for age group 15–19, education shows a stronger negative effect on female than on male fertility.

Figure 5.6 charts fertility patterns by education for age group 20–24. The trend line connecting the R_{ASFRs} for the illiterates is significantly lower than those representing other educational groups. This finding suggests that receiving education brings up the values of R_{ASFRs}, which is likely to be achieved by lowering female fertility to a greater extent than male fertility. A stronger inhibitive effect of education on female than on male fertility is again demonstrated for age group 20–24. However, when groups with different levels of education are considered, the effect of education on fertility does not seem to interact with sex in a clear manner considering the trend lines are mingled with each other for most years. So the general conclusion for age group 20–24 is that receiving education decreases female fertility to a greater extent than male fertility. Nevertheless, the level of education does not appear to differentiate male and female fertility.

I next show the R_{ASFRs} of six educational groups for age group 25–29 in Fig. 5.7. Clearly, besides the trend lines representing the illiterates and college/ university graduates, the trend lines for other educational groups all show a pattern of male fertility being higher than female fertility for most years. This pattern occurs because the peak of female fertility occurs in earlier years whereas male fertility begins to

Fig. 5.6 Ratios of male and female ASFRs by educational attainment for age group 20–24: Taiwan, 1974–2002 Sources: see sources for Fig. 5.1.

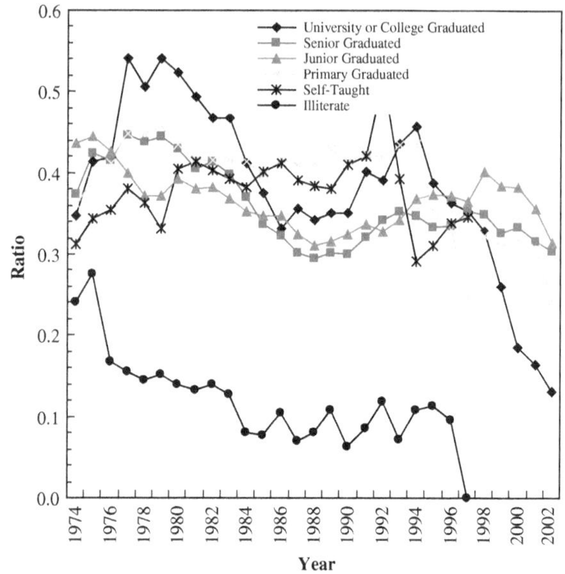

Fig. 5.7 Ratios of male and female ASFRs by educational attainment for age group 25–29: Taiwan, 1974–2002 Sources: see sources for Fig. 5.1.

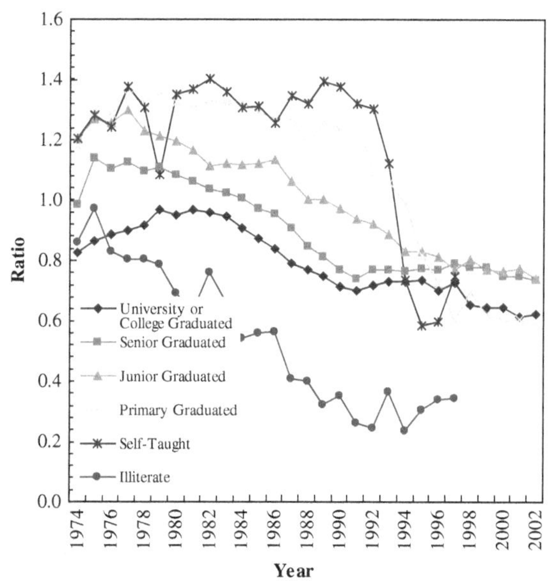

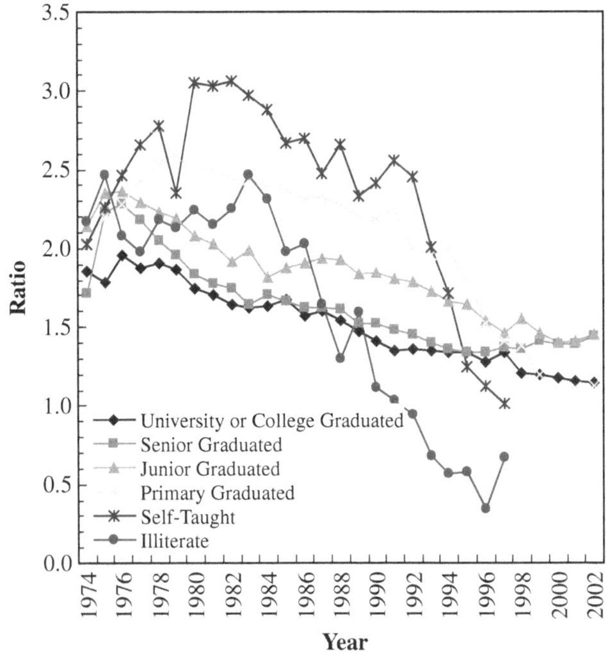

Fig. 5.8 Ratios of male and female ASFRs by educational attainment for age group 30–34: Taiwan, 1974–2002
Sources: see sources for Fig. 5.1.

reach its peak in this age group for most years studied. This age effect on fertility by sex may surpass the educational effect on differentiating male and female fertility. The effect of education on fertility by sex can be stated as follows: First, women with no education show a higher level of fertility than men, which offsets the age effect on fertility that has led to a higher male than female fertility shown in other educational groups. Second, for most years, especially for years prior to the early 1990s, education shows a stronger inhibitive effect on male than on female fertility. This is because the trend lines representing educational groups are laddered according to the level of education-the higher the level of education, the lower the values of R_{ASFRs}, the lower male as compared to female fertility. Recall findings from previous analysis that male fertility has become lower than female fertility since the late 1980s. The results shown here suggest that the lower male than female fertility could be caused by the increasing level of education for Taiwanese in recent decades.

The fertility pattern by sex and education for age group 30–34 is shown in Fig. 5.8. The ratios of male to female fertility for all educational groups in this chart are above 1.0, which could be mainly due to the age effect on male and female fertility. This is because men tend to have births in later ages than women. Thus, for this age group, the age effect on differentiating male and female fertility is stronger

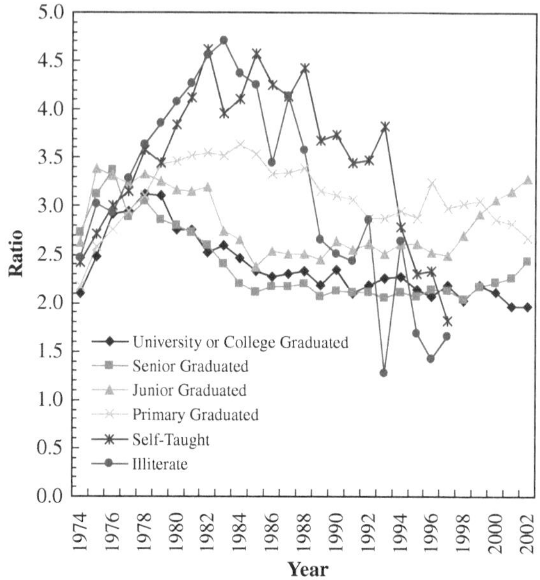

Fig. 5.9 Ratios of male and female ASFRs by educational attainment for age group 35–39: Taiwan, 1974–2002
Sources: see sources for Fig. 5.1.

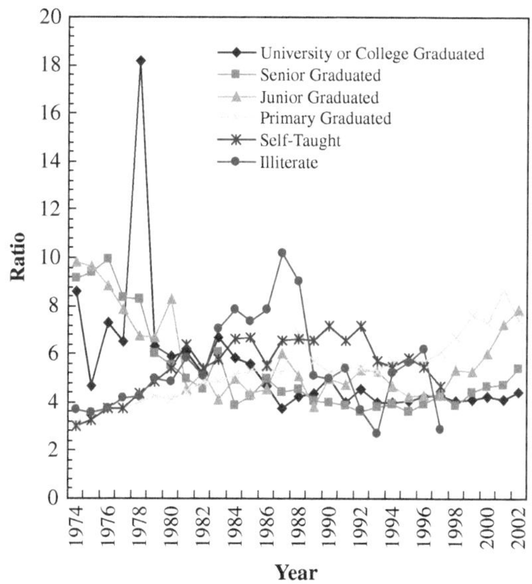

Fig. 5.10 Ratios of male and female ASFRs by educational attainment for age group 40–44: Taiwan, 1974–2002
Sources: see sources for Fig. 5.1.

than the educational effect in shaping fertility patterns by sex. Though there is a pattern that education decreases male fertility to a greater extent than female fertility, the trend lines for various educational groups tend to intertwine with each other. The effect of education on differentiating male and female fertility does not seem to be as clear as that for younger age groups.

The age-specific fertility by educational attainment for age group 35–39 is exhibited by Fig. 5.9. Male fertility is observed to be much higher than female fertility, considering the R_{ASFRs} values for all educational groups are above 1.0. This fertility pattern is again caused by the stronger age effect on male than on female fertility. The higher R_{ASFRs} values for illiterates and self-taught individuals during the late 1970s and the early 1990s demonstrate a stronger preventive effect of education on male than on female fertility.

Figures 5.10 and 5.11 plot the R_{ASFRs} by educational attainment for age groups 40–44 and 45–49, respectively. Compared to younger age groups, the R_{ASFRs} for each educational group is far above 1.0, suggesting a much higher male than female fertility. The trend lines for various educational groups intertwine with each other with fluctuations, which implies that education may no longer be a factor that distinguishes male and female age-specific fertility among individuals aged 40 and older.

To summarize the findings in this sub-section, educational attainment shapes fertility patterns by sex. For the youngest age group, 15–19, a higher level of education has a stronger negative effect on female than on male fertility. Moving to age group 20–24, the negative effect of education on fertility persists; however, the fertility differentials caused by level of education are not shown. The negative effect of education then becomes stronger on male than on female fertility starting from age group 25–29. I propose that the stronger preventive effect of education on male than on female age-specific fertility can be a factor that has caused male total fertility being lower than that of females in Taiwan in recent years. For age groups 30–34

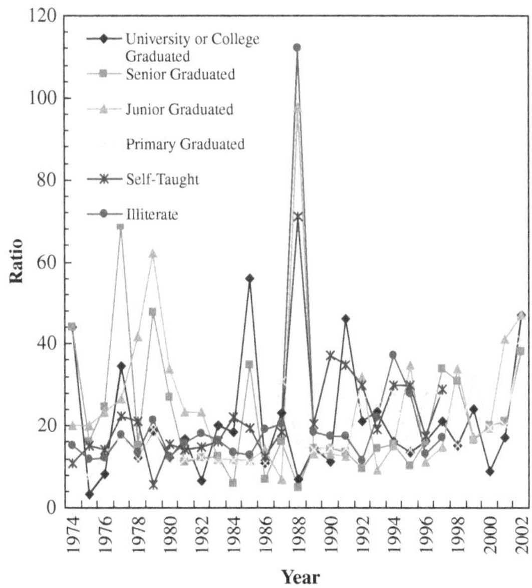

Fig. 5.11 Ratios of male and female ASFRs by educational attainment for age group 45–49: Taiwan, 1974–2002 Sources: see sources for Fig. 5.1.

and 35–39, compared to the effect of education, the age effect turns to be stronger than the educational effect on differentiating male and female fertility.

After age 40, the effect of education on distinguishing male and female fertility is no longer significant and is offset by the effect of age. Then why is the negative effect of education on female fertility stronger than on male fertility for people younger than 24 but the educational effect turns to be stronger on male than on female fertility for people in later ages? Anderson (1975) shows that education has a particular important effect on controlling fertility of women under age 30. This finding may have provided a possible explanation to the results shown in this research, that is, education plays a role in determining women's fertility in younger ages but the effect of education diminishes with age increasing. For males, the educational effect on fertility is less sensitive to age. Thus, the educational effect on female fertility is shown to be stronger than on male fertility in younger ages but the reverse pattern is the case in older ages.

Readers should be aware that results of this research are based on the analysis at the aggregate level. A variety of demographic, socioeconomic, cultural and political factors have not been controlled. Future research may need to extend the analysis to the individual level in order to explore the subject in a finer manner.

5.3.4 Male Fertility in Counties and Cities of Taiwan, 2002

I now turn to the final part of this study by examining male fertility in 23 counties and cities of Taiwan in year 2002. I intend to assess whether fertility theories that based on female fertility changes can be used to explain male fertility variation. The results of this part of the analysis answers the question raised in Chapter 1 that whether fertility theories based on females can well explain fertility of men. I start the analysis by describing male and female TFRs in 23 sub-regions in 2002, with detailed information shown in Table 5.2.

As it may be seen, in year 2002, most counties and cities have female fertility rates higher than their corresponding male fertility rates. Across the 23 subregions, females have a mean TFR value of 1,406 with a standard deviation of 211. They vary from a high of 1,845 in Hsinchu County to a low of 1,070 in Tainan City. Males have an average TFR value among the subregions of 1,330 with a standard deviation of 153. The highest male TFR is 1,705 in Hsinchu County and the lowest is 1,090 in Tainan City. The female mean TFR is higher than the male mean TFR by a difference of 76 births per 1,000 persons. Taipei County has the same male and female TFRs. Only a few subregions have higher male than female TFRs, namely, Taichung City, Chiayi City, Tainan City, the Taipei Municipality and the Kaohsiung Municipality. The results of the cross-sectional analysis support findings of the longitudinal analysis that female fertility in recent years has become higher than that of males.

Ordinary least squares (OLS) regression is then used to show the correlation of male and female fertility. The female TFRs are treated as an independent variable to predict male TFRs for the 23 subregions. The adjusted R^2 for this regression is 0.82,

Table 5.2 Male and female TFRs: 23 sub-regions of Taiwan, 2002

Sub-region	Abbreviation	Male	Female
Tainan city	KeC	1,610	1,710
Kaohsiung municipality	HsC	1,835	1,880
Taipei county	TacC	1,775	1,675
Chiayi city	ChC	1,605	1,640
Taipei municipality	TnC	1,545	1,550
Keelung city	TaiH	1,680	1,670
Taichung city	IlH	1,810	1,940
Kaohsiung county	TaoH	1,915	1,925
Tainan county	HsH	1,985	2,235
Ilan county	MiH	1,795	2,035
Taichung county	TacH	1,860	1,905
Pingtung county	ChaH	1,805	1,950
Hualien county	NaH	1,775	1,985
Taoyuan county	YuH	1,750	2,080
Penghu county	ChiH	1,690	2,035
Chaghwa county	TnH	1,605	1,785
Nantou county	KaoH	1,640	1,785
Hsinchu city	PinH	1,710	1,895
Taitung county	That	1,655	1,975
Yunlin county	HuaH	1,755	1,960
Mioali county	PeH	1,505	1,750
Chiayi county	TaiM	1,495	1,415
Hsinchu county	KaoM	1,515	1,515

Source: *Taiwan-Fukien Demographic Fact Book* 2002.

indicating that more than 80% of the variance in male fertility may be explained by female fertility. This finding indicates that male and female fertility rates are highly correlated with each other.

I further plot the residuals from the above regression equation (vertical axis) by values of male TFRs (horizontal axis) in Fig. 5.12. Subregions below the line have predicted values of male fertility larger than their actual values and subregions above the line have predicted values smaller than their actual values. Results show that the error using female TFRs to predict male TFRs increases with increasing values of male fertility. This finding falls in line with findings of the previous chapter that male and female fertility differentials increase with an increasing value of TFR.

Given that I intend to address the demographic concern that whether existing fertility theories can explain male fertility variation, in this sub-section of the chapter, I apply several theoretical models based on female fertility changes to predict fertility of men among subregions of Taiwan in 2002. Some theoretical frameworks applied in this research are first reviewed below.

Educational attainment and fertility decline perspective. A consistently negative relationship between education and fertility has been found in Taiwan by many scholars (Chang, Freedman & Sun, 1987; Hermalin, 1974; Li, 1973). It has been

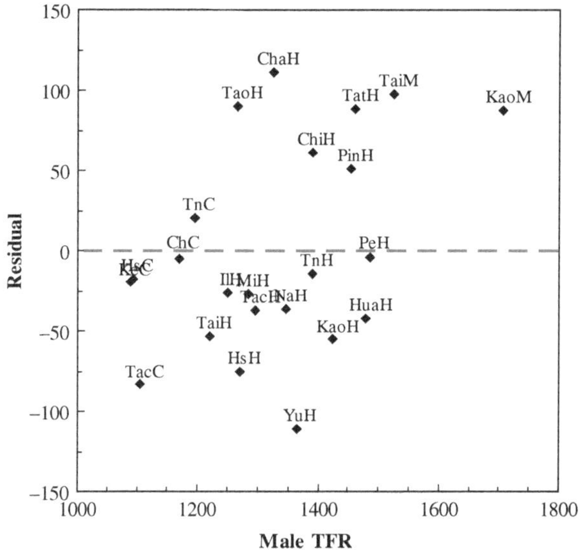

Fig. 5.12 Residuals vs. male TFRs: 23 counties and cities of Taiwan, 2002
Sources: see sources for Table 5.2. Abbreviated versions of names for counties and cities are used here. For full names, see Table 5.2.

revealed that fertility differentials caused by education are greater than fertility differentials caused by other factors, such as the rural-urban differences (Chang et al., 1987, p. 326). When the age effect is also taken into consideration, prior research shows that educational attainment is particularly important in controlling fertility of women under age 30 (Anderson, 1975). Previous analyses also show that the negative effect of education on fertility can be applied not only to Taiwanese females in general, but also to the married individuals in particular (Freedman, Fan, Wei, & Weinberger, 1977). Moreover, the effect of education on fertility is found to vary across different educational groups. It has been reported that "while structural changes in educational level have had a significant effect in producing lower fertility in Taiwan, the major effects come from changes in fertility within educational strata; fertility has declined especially rapidly among the more poorly educated strata" (Freedman et al., 1977, p. 18). Based on these findings, researchers claim that education is "the most important factor affecting fertility attitudes and behavior" of Taiwanese women (Speare, Speare, & Lin, 1973, p. 333).

Socioeconomic change and fertility reduction approach. The second theoretical framework examines fertility reduction in Taiwan from the perspective of socioeconomic changes. Researchers view social and economic development as an aggregate setting that has influenced female fertility decline. Economic welfare, such as family income, along with general health conditions, particularly as reflected in infant mortality rate, are observed to be negatively related to fertility (Li, 1973; Muller & Cohn, 1977). Some other socioeconomic factors are also shown to reduce birth rates indirectly through mediating with family planning programs and other variables more proximate to fertility (Poston and Dudley, 2000). As Poston (Poston and Dudley, 2000, p. 57) writes, "[in Taiwan], there were strong influences of social and economic development factors on fertility." Other researchers also conclude that some dimensions indicating socioeconomic changes, such as urbanization, a rising age at marriage, and the diffusion effects of mass media have played a decisive role in reducing Taiwanese' fertility (Chang et al., 1987; Hermalin, 1974; Li, 1973).

Other explanations. Besides the above approaches, previous studies have also suggested the importance of preferred family size and family planning programs in influencing female fertility changes in Taiwan (Chang et al., 1987; Freedman et al., 1977; Hermalin, 1974; Jejeebhoy, 1981). Despite female labor force participation has long been used as a predictor of fertility decline (Smith-Lovin & Tickamyer, 1978; Terry, 1975; Waite & Stolzenberg, 1976), in Taiwan, this variable has been found to be only weakly related to reproductive behavior. Unpaid family workers do not seem to display higher fertility than those in the market sector (Stokes & Hsieh, 1983).

The above reviewed theoretical frameworks provide guidance to this current research. Due to data constraint, I will test mainly the applicability of educational and socioeconomic approaches on male fertility. I reserve most comments on the effects of other dimensions that can possibly influence fertility for later in this book. Variables that represent educational and socioeconomic dimensions are used to predict both male and female fertility in the regression models. I contrast the regression results for the male and female models in order to assess the efficacy of these two fertility theories when predicting male fertility. The measures that represent the educational and socioeconomic dimensions are as follows: (1) percent of males and females who were receiving or have received college degrees in 1997; (2) combined average family income in 1998; (3) infant mortality rate in 1997; (4) percentages of married males and females in age group 20–24 in 1997; and (5) population density (per square kilometer) in 1997. Table 5.3 presents the descriptive statistics for these independent variables.

Variation is observed in each of these five independent variables. Average combined family income, for instance, ranges from NT$660,563 in Penghu County to NT$1,531,961 in Taipei Municipality, and population density ranges from 532 people per square kilometer in Taitung County to 131, 635 people per square kilometer in Kaohsiung Municipality. Because high collinearity occurs among some independent variables, three OLS regressions are estimated to model male and female TFRs. The OLS regression results predicting male and female fertility are presented in Tables 5.4 and 5.5, respectively. For all regression models, unstandardized and standardized regression coefficients are reported for each independent variable. The sign of "–" indicates that a particular variable is omitted in the regression model due to high collinearity.

According to results displayed in both tables, for Model 1, education has a significantly negative effect on both male and female fertility, controlling for the effects of other independent variables (see significant regression coefficients in both tables).

Table 5.3 Descriptive statistics for fertility rates and independent variables: 23 counties and cities of Taiwan

Variable	Mean	S.D.	Min. value	Max. value
Dependent variable				
Male TFR	1,330.0	152.6	1,090.0, Tainan city	1,705.0, Hsinchu county
Female TFR	1,406.7	211.3	1,070.0, Tainan city	1,845.0, Hsinchu county
Independent variable				
% male received/ receiving college degree	9.4	3.9	3.2, Taoyuan county	18.8, Taipei municipality
% female received/ receiving college degree	9.2	3.0	5.2, Taitung county	17.5, Taipei municipality
Average combined family income (NT$)	1,017,699.0	203,255.8	660,563.0, Penghu county	1,531,961.0, Taipei municipality
Infant mortality rate	7.5	1.2	6.1, Taitung county	10.8, Hualien county
% married males in age group 20–24	21.0	5.2	2.6, Taipei municipality	8.9, Yunlin county
% married females in age group 20–24	6.3	1.7	9.4, Taipei municipality	28.0, Taitung county
Population density per sq. km. of cultivated area	15,392.4	30,959.3	532.0, Taitung county	131,635.0, Kaohsiung municipality
N = 23				

1 U.S. dollar = NT$34.58 in July 2002, and NT$31.6 in 1998. *The World Fact Book.*
Sources: *Taiwan-Fuchiun Demographic Fact Book* 1997, Tables 6, 7, 8, 10 and 39; *Republic of China National Statistics*, 1998.

Together, the three variables account for 10% of male fertility variation and 23% of female fertility changes. A higher R-squared value for the female model than for the male model suggests that Model 1 predicts female fertility better than it does on male fertility.

For Model 2 in both tables, the education variable is replaced by a variable measuring the percentage of males (or females) in age group 20–24 who are married. This variable represents the socioeconomic level of a society. The rationale behind this variable is that the higher the socioeconomic level of a society, the later the age at marriage. Thus, a higher percentage of males or females being married for age group 20–24 indicates a relatively lower socioeconomic level. According to results shown in Model 2, the marriage variable has the most sizable effect on both male and female fertility. The three variables in Model 2 together account for 75% of the variation in female fertility as compared to 51% of the variation in male fertility. These findings again show that the model explains female fertility better than male fertility.

Table 5.4 Multiple regression coefficients for male TFRs: 23 counties and cities of Taiwan, 2002

	Model 1		Model 2		Model 3	
Independent variable	Unstandardized	Standardized	Unstandardized	Standardized	Unstandardized	Standardized
Average combined family income	0.00	0.20	0.00**	0.58**	0.00	0.21
Infant mortality rate	−1.87	−0.01	−25.44	−0.19	−1.43	−0.01
% males received college degree	−21.50*	−0.56*	–	–	–	–
% married males in age group 20–24	–		94.50***	1.05***	–	–
Pop. density per sq. km. of cultivated area	–		–	–	−0.00*	−0.60*
Constant	1,394.25		482.21		1,225.53	
R^2 (adjusted)	0.10		0.51		0.16	
df	19		19		19	
N = 23						

*$p < 0.05$, **$p < 0.01$, ***$p < 0.001$ (two-tailed test).

Table 5.5 Multiple regression coefficients for female TFRs: 23 counties and cities of Taiwan, 2002

	Model 1		Model 2		Model 3	
Independent variable	Unstandardized	Standardized	Unstandardized	Standardized	Unstandardized	Standardized
Average combined family income	−0.00	−0.18	0.00*	0.34*	−0.00	−0.20
Infant mortality rate	8.37	0.05	−34.15	−0.19	12.12	0.07
% females received/receiving college degree	−31.48*	−0.44*	–	–	–	–
Percent married females in age group 20–24	–		46.71***	1.15***	–	–
Pop. density per sq. km. of cultivated area	–		–	–	– 0.00*	−0.47*
Constant	1,826.84		316.10		1,580.50	
R^2 (adjusted)	0.23		0.74		0.28	
df	19		19		19	
N = 23						

$^{*}p < 0.05$, $^{**}p < 0.01$, $^{***}p < 0.001$ (two-tailed test).

The last columns of Tables 5.4 and 5.5 show the results of multiple regression equations in which the population density variable replaces the percent married variable. As expected, the population density variable demonstrates a negative effect on both male and female fertility rates. Its influence on fertility is also stronger than those of the other two variables in the models, namely, family income and infant mortality. Again, the combined effect of the three variables in Model 3 is stronger for female fertility than for male fertility.

Overall, the results of the three models that regress male and female fertility show many similarities. Specifically, the infant mortality variable and the economic development indicator of *combined family income* are not significant, whereas the education and marriage variables are significant and influential. In fact, the marriage variable is found to be the most significant factor influencing both male and female fertility. Thus, the model that contains the marriage variable has the strongest explanatory capability than other models. The urbanization indicator *population density* is shown to be negatively associated with male and female fertility.

These findings suggest that despite fertility theories account for male and female fertility variation in a similar manner, there is significant variance in male fertility that cannot be explained by current fertility theories based on females.

5.4 Discussion and Summary

In this chapter, I have focused closely on Taiwan and have examined male fertility in rates as compared to female fertility in this specific locale. The chapter begins by examining male and female TFRs in Taiwan for years 1975–2004. It is revealed that male and female fertility rates for most years were not identical. In earlier years, male TFRs were higher than female TFRs, and the reverse pattern was true since the late 1980s. Cross-sectionally, male and female fertility are shown to differ among the 23 subregions of Taiwan in 2002, with female fertility surpassing male fertility in most subregions. These findings are consistent with that reached in the previous chapter, that is, with the TFR declines below the replacement level, male fertility turns to be lower than female fertility.

The second major finding of this chapter is that the age-specific fertility also differs by sex in Taiwan. The age-specific fertility patterns generally fall in line with those found in other industrialized countries (see Chapter 4), with significant fertility differentials showing at age groups 45–49 and over. Additionally, my analysis demonstrates a critical role of education in shaping age-specific fertility by sex. Briefly, for age group 15–19, education has a stronger negative effect on female than on male fertility. The negative influence of education then turns to be stronger on men's childbearing outcome from ages 25–39. Conventional demography has focused a great deal on the importance of educational attainment on deterring female fertility. This analysis, however, shows that at the aggregate level, education can deter male fertility to a greater extent as compared to female fertility in certain ages. Based on these findings, I argue that the stronger preventive effect of education on male than on female age-specific fertility in middle age groups can be a factor that has caused male total fertility being lower than that of females in recent years. After age 40, education is no longer a factor distinguishing male and female fertility.

The explanation of the age-specific fertility differentials by sex is perhaps more complex than what is shown here, which involves socioeconomic changes, family planning programs, development of modern contraceptive methods, changing views of women's role in society and increasing rates of marital disruption. Future research may need to incorporate a variety of factors to investigate fertility differentials by sex to improve this current analysis.

In addition to the above findings, I have addressed the demographic concern that whether existing fertility theories based on females can account for the dynamics of male fertility. The results do suggest some similarities between models that regress male and female fertility. Particularly, the socioeconomic and educational variables show similar influence on men's and women's fertility outcomes, with the marriage variable showing the most significant effect on fertility for both sexes. Nonetheless, the regression models perform better when predicting female fertility than male fertility. These results suggest that there are likely other factors that need to be introduced into the equations, which influence male fertility but have heretofore not been considered. I will attempt to explore these factors at the individual level in the following chapters.

References

Anderson, B. A. (1975). Male age and fertility results from Ireland prior to 1911. *Population Index*, *41*(4), 561–567.

Chang, M. C., Freedman, R., & Sun, T. H. (1987). Trends in fertility, family size preferences, and family planning practices in Taiwan, 1961-85. *Studies in Family Planning*, *18*(6), 320–337.

Collver, A., Speare, A. J., & Liu, P. K. C. (1967). Local variations of fertility in Taiwan. *Population Studies*, *20*(3), 329–342.

Freedman, R., Fan, T. H., Wei, S. P., & Weinberger, M. B. (1977). Trends in fertility and in the effects of education on fertility in Taiwan. *Studies in Family Planning*, *8*(1), 11–18.

Hermalin, A. (1974). Empirical research in Taiwan on factors underlying differences in fertility. *Studies in Family Planning*, *5*(10), 314–324.

Jejeebhoy, S. J. (1981). Cohort consistency in family size preferences: Taiwan, 1965–73. *Studies in Family Planning*, *12*(5), 229–232.

Li, W. L. (1973). Temporal and spatial analysis of fertility decline in Taiwan. *Population Studies*, *27*(1), 97–104.

The Ministry of the Interior of Republic of China (2002). *Taiwan-Fukien demographic fact book.* Taipei: Ministry of the Interior of Republic of China.

The Ministry of the Interior of the Republic of China (2005). *Taiwan-Fukien demographic fact book.* Taipei: The Ministry of the Interior of Republic of China.

Muller, E. & Cohn, R. (1977). The relation of income to fertility decisions in Taiwan. *Economic Development and Cultural Change*, *25*(2), 325–347.

Poston, D. L. (2000). Social and economic development and the fertility transitions in mainland China and Taiwan. *Population and Development Review*, *26*(Supplement), 40–60.

Smith-Lovin, L. & Tickamyer, A. R. (1978). Nonrecursive models of labor force participation, fertility behavior and sex role attitudes. *American Sociological Review*, *43*(4), 541–557.

Speare, A., Speare, M. C., & Lin, H. S. (1973). Urbanization, non-familial work, education and fertility in Taiwan. *Population Studies*, *27*(2), 323–334.

Stokes, C. S. & Hsieh, Y. S. (1983). Female employment and reproductive behavior in Taiwan, 1980. *Demography*, *20*(3), 313–331.

Terry, G. B. (1975). Rival explanations in the work-fertility relationship. *Population Studies*, *28*(2), 191–205.

Waite, L. J. & Stolzenberg, R. M. (1976). Intended childbearing and labor force participation of young women: Insights from nonrecursive models. *American Sociological Review*, *41*(2), 235–251.

Part III
Male and Female Fertility Differentials in Determinants

Chapter 6
Demographic, Socioeconomic Characteristics, and Male and Female Fertiltiy

Demographers for many decades have documented that female fertility differentials result from demographic and socioeconomic differentiation. Most often investigated are female fertility differences across racial and ethnic groups (Forste & Tienda, 1996; Wildsmith & Raley, 2006). The U.S. foreign-born population has also been shown to have a higher fertility than their U.S.-born counterparts (Bean, Swicegood, & Berg, 2000; Johnson, 1979; Kahn, 1994). Other demographic variables, such as age, metropolitan residence and marriage also show significant effects on female fertility (Burnight, Whetten, & Waxman, 1956; Lavely, 1986; Zeng, Vaupel, & Yashin, 1985). In addition to these demographic factors, socioeconomic variables, including education, income and employment have been found crucial as well when determining female fertility (Borg, 1989; Budig, 2003; Dreze & Murthi, 2001).

The correlation between demographic and socioeconomic characteristics and men's fertility, however, has not been fully explored. In large part, this is because data on male fertility are often unavailable or of poor quality. Using fertility data of the NSFG Cycle 6, this chapter documents and examines the influence of a variety of demographic and socioeconomic factors on male fertility. These factors are such as age, racial and ethnic composition, nativity, metropolitan residence, marriage, education, income and labor force participation, which are considered as central measures in the construction of demographic and socioeconomic characteristics. I evaluate how the effects of these demographic and socioeconomic variables on fertility vary by gender. In this chapter and the following chapters, I use the word "gender" rather than "sex" because the determinants of fertility are more social in orientation. The results of this chapter and the following chapters enlighten the reader the manner in which this research helps to construct fertility theories of men. Findings of this analysis also provide policy implications for existing family planning programs.

L. Zhang, *Male Fertility Patterns and Determinants*, The Springer Series on Demographic Methods and Population Analysis 27, DOI 10.1007/978-90-481-8939-7_6,

6.1 Linking Demographic Characteristics to Fertility

A variety of demographic factors have been found influential in determining fertility outcome. Among demographic variables, age has been consistently shown in the literature to be correlated with women's overall fertility in a positive manner. It is suggested that this relationship is due to older women having been in childbearing status for a longer period of time than younger women (Coale & Trussell, 1974; Wood & Weinstein, 1988; Xie & Pimentel, 1992). As for men, the age effect on overall fertility has not been empirically tested. Studies have mainly presented a picture of male fertility being less restricted by age than female fertility. For instance, Mineau and Trussell (1982) examine the age patterns of the nineteenth century Mormons' fertility and find that the age effect on husband's total fertility is not as strong as that on wife's fertility. The analysis of Goldman and Montgomery (1989) also reveals that before age 35, male aging has little influence on their fertility outcome. These findings, however, do not necessarily suggest that age does not have an effect on male overall fertility. Instead, I expect that age has a stronger effect on men's overall fertility than on that of women. I believe this to be the case because women start their childbearing earlier and they have a shorter reproductive span compared to men. Ages 15–49 are typically women's childbearing ages (Coale & Tye, 1961; Lavely, 1986), whereas the reproductive ages of men continue to their 70 s (Keyfitz, 1977). Men's longer reproductive span and later fertility peak should eventually lead to a stronger cumulative effect of age on male fertility than on female fertility. On the basis of this rationale, my hypotheses predict the age effects on male and female fertility are as follows:

Hypothesis 1: Age has a positive effect on both men's and women's fertility, controlling for other factors. But,

Hypothesis 2: The effect of age on male fertility is stronger than that on female fertility.

Besides age, demographers have also documented fertility differentials across U.S. racial and ethnic groups. Most often investigated is fertility of Caucasians, Latinos and African Americans. Women of Hispanic origin have been found to exhibit a distinctively higher level of fertility than those of any other racial or ethnic group, followed by African American women (Aneshensel, Fielder, & Becerra, 1989; Forste & Tienda, 1996; Johnson, 1979; Saenz & Morales, 2005). Caucasian women along with Asian women are observed to have the lowest fertility rates in the U.S. (Saenz & Morales, 2005). A number of perspectives have been proposed to elucidate the fertility differentials across racial and ethnic groups. Some demographers argue that the pronatalist cultural norms of Latin countries and the recently increased number of Latino immigrants have resulted in a higher fertility rate for Latino women. Others contend that the white-black community environment differences have caused the white–black fertility differentials. This is because different racial and ethnic communities have formed different views towards childbearing and marriage, which is a key factor that determines fertility variation among women with diverse racial and ethnic backgrounds (Forste & Tienda, 1996; Saenz, 2004; South & Baumer, 2000).

Limited research has been done regarding male fertility differentials across race and ethnicity. Bachu's (1996) study does exhibit a higher fertility of men with Hispanic origin as compared to men with other racial and ethnic backgrounds. However, fertility differences of men among Caucasians, Blacks and the rest of the other racial and ethnic groups remain unexplored. As far as the comparison of male and female fertility outcomes due to race and ethnicity, Bachu points out that there are minimal differences in fertility between men and women across race and ethnicity among married American couples. For never-married population, Bachu shows that gender differences in fertility do exist with black women having a significantly higher level of fertility than black men. In other words, being black has a stronger positive effect on female than on male fertility. From this stand point of view, I expect race and ethnicity to interact with gender when shaping fertility outcome. Thus, my next two hypotheses are set forth as follows:

Hypothesis 3: Racial and ethnic differences in fertility are present among both men and women, controlling for other factors. But,

Hypothesis 4: The fertility differentials caused by an individual's racial and ethnic composition varies by gender.

In addition to the fertility differences across racial and ethnic groups, it is revealed that the U.S. foreign-born population has a higher level of fertility than their U.S. born counterparts (Bean et al., 2000; Hervitz, 1985; Jaffe & Cullen, 1975; Kahn, 1994; Singley & Landale, 1998). Researchers argue that it is because the majority of the foreign-born population comes from economically-disadvantaged societies with high-fertility norms and traditions (Stephen & Bean, 1992). The high-fertility norms and traditions have stimulated women's childbearing behavior. Such a positive influence of foreign nativity on fertility has been found applicable to the U.S. males as well. For instance, Bachu (1996) reveals that foreign-born husbands have a higher fertility than native-born husbands. Bachu further shows that foreign-born husbands' fertility is especially high when they are married to foreign-born wives. The gender differences in the association of nativity and fertility, nevertheless, has not been documented in prior literature. Based on these findings, I propose the following hypotheses for testing:

Hypothesis 5: Being foreign-born has a positive effect on both male and female fertility, controlling for other factors. And,

Hypothesis 6: The impact of nativity on fertility does not vary by gender.

In the literature of fertility, residence is also shown to influence people's childbearing behavior. Generally, urban residents display a relatively lower level of fertility than their rural counterparts; people living in central cities tend to have fewer children than people on fringes of metropolitan areas (Burnight et al., 1956; Goldstein & Mayer, 1965; Okore, 1980). This residential effect on fertility has been considered as a consequence of delayed childbearing and the preference for a smaller family size during the processes of urbanization and modernization (Robinson, 1963; Zeng & Vaupel, 1989). When it comes to the correlation between residence and male fertility, it has been shown that men living in central cities have higher childlessness rates than their counterparts who live in suburban or non-metropolitan areas (Bachu, 1996). Prior literature has not shown significant gender differences in the relationship of place of residence and fertility. According to these result, I expect that urban residence decreases men's fertility as it does on female fertility. According to these findings, my hypotheses regarding residence and fertility are as follows:

Hypothesis 7: Residing in urban settings decreases the level of fertility for both men and women, controlling for other factors. And,

Hypothesis 8: Residential fertility differences do not vary by gender.

The last demographic characteristic that will be discussed here is marital status. A positive association between being married and women's childbearing has been repeatedly found in the literature (Bongaarts, 1982; Sanchez, 1998; Zeng et al., 1985). Researchers also find that the majority of births occur in marital unions although increased non-marital fertility has been recently witnessed in the U.S. and other industrialized nations (Mosher, Johnson, & Horn, 1986). Discussions that directly address the influence of marital status on men's fertility are rarely seen in the literature. A few studies may have provided evidence to link marriage and male and female fertility differentials through emphasizing the interruption effect of marriage on people's educational career. Studies show that marriage interrupts both men's and women's educational career, with marriage being more detrimental to women's educational careers than men's (Alexander & Reilly, 1981; Teachman & Polonko, 1988). Given education has a negative effect on both men's and women's fertility, if I link marriage, education and fertility together, then I would hypothesize that marriage has a stronger positive effect on female than on male fertility when marriage mediates with people's educational achievements. The rationale behind this hypothesis is that since marriage has a stronger negative effect on women's educational career and lower education is usually treated as a stimulus to fertility (the negative association between education and fertility will be discussed in the following subsection of this chapter), then marriage is likely to increase women's fertility to a greater extent than men's fertility. On the basis of the above rationale, I state the following two hypotheses:

Hypothesis 9: With everything else being equal, marriage increases both men's and women's fertility. But,

Hypothesis 10: Marriage should have a stronger positive effect on female than on male fertility, controlling for other factors.

6.2 Previous Literature on Socioeconomic Characteristics and Fertility

Socioeconomic status is also a primary determinant of fertility. Its effect is often discussed and assessed by examining factors such as education, income, and occupational prestige. These factors will be treated as major measures of socioeconomic status in this study. In terms of the correlation between education and fertility, previous studies have generally documented a negative association between education and female fertility (Anderson, 1975; Jain, 1981; London, 1992; van de Walle, 1980; Weinberger, 1987), although a positive relationship is also found in less-developed countries at the lower end of the educational range (Martin, 1995). Researchers argue that the major mechanisms that enable education to depress female fertility include, enhancement of women's power to make reproductive choices, an increase in women's contraceptive use, a delayed age at marriage, and an increased female labor force participation rate which reduces women's time for childbearing (Anderson, 1975; Cameron, Dowling, & Worswick, 2001; Martin, 1995; Rindfuss, Morgan, & Offutt, 1996; Weinberger, 1987). Prior research has also revealed a number of channels through which education may influence women's childbearing behavior. For instance, Kravdal (2002) points out that educational achievements at the aggregate level interact with an individual's fertility behavior at the micro level. As Kravdal shows, a higher average educational level in a community inhibits an individual woman's childbearing behavior. A study conducted by Skirbekk and colleagues (2004) reveals that education influences women's fertility through affecting women's timing of marriage so that it affects women's childbearing behavior. Researchers further indicate that education may influence fertility through medicating with a number of other factors. For example, Rindfuss and colleagues (1980) show that the relationship between education and fertility depends on a woman's age at first birth. They emphasize that once the process of childbearing has started, education begins to have an indirect effect on fertility through mediating with age at first birth.

As to men, previous studies have also provided some evidence with regard to the correlation between their schooling and fertility. For example, my analysis of Taiwanese fertility has documented a negative association between education and male fertility. The negative effect of education on male fertility is found to be not as strong as on that of women's fertility for certain age groups (see Chapter 5). Through analyzing data from 20 countries participating in the World Fertility Surveys (WFS), Rodrigues and Cleland (1981) show similar findings. In Europe, researchers have also conducted a series of studies examining male and female transitions to adulthood in 24 countries using survey data for the 1980s and 1990s. Their research confirms the results of previous analyses that education appears to have a stronger preventive effect on female than on male fertility. According to these results, I expect education to be more influential in decreasing women's than men's fertility, with everything else being equal. Thus, my next two hypotheses are proposed as follows:

Hypothesis 11: Education has a negative correlation with both men's and women's fertility, controlling for other factors. However,

Hypothesis 12: The depressing effect of education on female fertility is stronger than that on male fertility.

Other than education, family income has been found to be one of the principal socioeconomic factors that shape fertility. Previous research shows inconsistent findings regarding the effect of income on fertility based on analyzing macro-level data. Some studies exhibit that family income is positively related to fertility (Ben-Porath, 1973; Easterlin, 1973). Others reveal that there is a reverse relationship between these two; an increased family income is indeed one of the causes of fertility decline (Freedman & Thornto, 1982; Li, 1973; Muller & Cohn, 1977; Poston & Dudley, 2000). Studies analyzing micro-data seem to support the latter, suggesting that family income reduces female fertility (Thornto, 1978; Westoff & Ryder, 1977). Borg (1989) attempts to resolve the discrepancy by arguing that the negative effect of income on fertility is in fact disguised by some other factors such as the net price of a child, the opportunity cost of the wife's time and supply factors, that play a role in the income and fertility relation. Once these factors are controlled, the effect of income on female fertility is positive and significant.

In terms of the income effect on male fertility, previous studies seem to provide evidence of a stronger positive effect of family income on male than on female fertility. Freedman and Thornto (1982) show that the husband's income is positively related to family size. Butz and Ward (1979) suggest that women's income is negatively related to their childbearing, with the opposite for men's income and fertility. Based on these findings, I hypothesize the following:

Hypothesis 13: Family income has a positive effect on both men's and women's fertility, controlling for other factors. But,

Hypothesis 14: Family income has a stronger positive effect on male than on female fertility.

Occupational prestige is another crucial indicator of socioeconomic status. In this research, instead of using occupational prestige to operationalize socioeconomic status, I apply a variable that represents an individual's employment status to examine the impact of socioeconomic status on fertility. I use this variable because previous literature has documented a strong correlation between employment and women's fertility. In general, prior studies show that increasing women's labor force participation leads to a fertility decline (Devaney, 1983; Lehrer & Nerlove, 1986; Rodrigues & Cleland, 1981; Smith-Lovin & Tickamyer, 1978; Waite & Stolzenberg, 1976). Two major theories have been proposed to account for this inverse relationship. The role incompatibility theory argues that mother and worker roles are not compatible in a modern society with an industrialized economy. This is because the bureaucratic occupational structure in such a society does not allow the flexibility required by childbearing. Moreover, the nuclear family system leaves women no alternatives but to take on the entire burden caring for children themselves (Smith-Lovin & Tickamyer, 1978; Watkins, 1986). As a result, women who participate in the labor force end up having fewer children. The microeconomic approach explains this inverse relationship from a cost/benefit point of view. According to this approach, with the rise in the economic costs of childbearing and the opportunity costs for being a mother, the benefits associated with working such as income and prestige outweigh the costs associated with childbearing. Consequently, women choose to have fewer children (Easterlin, 1973; Mincer, 1963) and fertility at the societal level declines.

Though the above proposed fertility theories have not been used to account for male fertility changes, a few studies have attempted to shed light on the influence of employment on men's fertility by contrasting men's and women's entry into parenthood. Martin and Stanfors (2006) show that there is a negative association between employment and maternity but a positive association between employment and paternity. Studies of unemployment and parenthood transition in other European countries also suggest that the effect of unemployment is gender-specific. Unemployment leads to men's postponement of marriage, whereas it affects women in two distinct ways. It either accelerates or slows down women's timing of marriage (Corijn & Klijzing, 2001). In line with the above findings, I predict employment status has a similar impact on male completed fertility as on their paternity, that is:

Hypothesis 15: Labor force participation has significantly different effects on male and female fertility, with a negative effect on female fertility but a positive effect on male fertility.

In the following sub-sections of the chapter, I will test my hypotheses by exploring the link between demographic and socioeconomic characteristics and male and female fertility, with a particular focus on highlighting the gender differences in such a link.

6.3 Data, Measures and Methods

This chapter uses data from the 2002 National Survey of Family Growth (NSFG) Cycle 6 to conduct the analysis. As already noted in a previous chapter (Chapter 3), the NSFG Cycle 6 was conducted by National Center for Health Statistics (NCHS) since 1973. For the previous five cycles, the NSFG questionnaires were geared merely towards women. Year 2002 was the first time that the NSFG included men in its surveys. Based on an area probability sampling strategy, 7,643 women and 4,928, 15–45 years of age, were included in NSFG Cycle 6 as nationally representative samples of the U.S. population. These samples were interviewed on topics of "fertility, marriage, cohabitation, contraception and related issues" (National Center for Health Statistics, 2005, p. 5).

As far as the topic of fertility is concerned, both male and female respondents were asked their fertility outcomes and history. The most important measure of male fertility that can be drawn from the Cycle 6 dataset is number of biological children born to the male respondent. The survey question that acquires this information is "how many biological children have you ever had?" Demographers often refer this measure to children ever born (CEB). An equivalent survey question regarding women's CEB is also presented in the Cycle 6 questionnaire. The question asks the female respondent "how many live births have you ever had?" These two questions are considered as the measuring tool of the dependent variable of this study, that is, men's and women's CEB.

In addition to these two fertility measures, the dataset also contains numerous covariates that are considered to be influential on fertility, which will be built into the analysis. Since I am also interested in investigating the gender differences in the link between a variety of demographic and socioeconomic factors and fertility, I combine two separate male and female NSFG datasets together into one data file. In the combined dataset, I create a gender variable which is coded as "1" if the respondent is a male and "0" if otherwise. By doing so, female respondents are set as the reference group in the analysis. I then multiply the independent variables with the gender variable to generate a series of gender interaction terms, which are used to test whether significant gender differences exist in the models estimating fertility.

The measures of demographic characteristics in this analysis include age, race and ethnicity, nativity, metropolitan residence and marriage which are considered as the central measures of the demographic composition. The variable *age* is coded as a continuous variable, ranging from 15 to 44 for females and 15 to 45 for males. The respondent's *race and ethnicity* is measured via categorizing the respondent into one of the following four racial and ethnic categories: Hispanics, non-Hispanic Whites, Blacks, and other racial and ethnic groups, including Asian and Pacific Islanders. Non-Hispanic Whites are set as the reference category. *Nativity* is a dummy variable which is coded as "1" if the respondent is foreign born and "0" if otherwise. *Residence* is coded as a set of dummy variables, including central city in Metropolitan Statistical Areas (MSAs), other non-central city areas in MSAs, and areas in non-MSAs. The group of respondents who resided in central cities of MSAs is considered as the reference group since they comprise nearly half of the total respondents for this particular variable. *Marriage* is often measured by current marital status of the respondent, that is, by placing the respondent into one of the following categories: married, never married (single), divorced/separate, and widowed. Given that the dependent variable, CEB, is a measure of completed fertility, current marital status may not be able to capture the influence of marriage on the respondent's fertility during a lifetime. In the NSFG dataset, there is another measure that describes the respondent's marital status by asking whether the respondent had ever been married. I did not choose this measure either due to the same concern. Thus, in my analysis, I use *number of times the respondent had married* as the marriage variable to examine the marriage effect on fertility. This is a continuous variable, which ranges from 0 to 4 for men and 0 to 5 for women.

As to measures of socioeconomic factors, I use the highest degree received to represent the respondent's *educational attainment*. In this dataset, respondents are categorized into four groups according to their educational attainments, which are: respondents with no diploma, respondents with high school degrees or less, respondents who received college degrees or some college degrees, and respondents with university degrees or above. *Income* is usually measured in multiple ways. It can be measured by individual or family income. For either one, it can be treated as a continuous or dichotomous variable. Some people also use the logged form of income to avoid a skewed distribution of income for a population. In this study, I choose family income to represent the income variable. The variable is measured by total combined gross family income in 2001, which is coded by the NSFG into 14 categories, varying from under $5,000 to $75,000 or more. In the analysis, I recode the values for the family income variable into four categories for the sake of simplicity. Those categories are: under $25,000, $25,000–$49,999, $50,000–$74,999 and $75,000 and over. People who had family income more than $75,000 in 2001 are defined as the reference category.

There are also multiple measures representing employment status. For example, people can be classified into categories of currently working, unemployed, or not in the labor force. Since I am interested in examining how labor force participation plays a role in determining fertility, the ideal measure of employment ought to represent an employment status that occurs before the childbearing behavior took place. In the NSFG dataset, the variable *ever worked full time for more than 6 months* appears to be the best measure. I therefore decided to use this measure to represent employment status, which is coded as "1" if the respondent who had ever worked for more than 6 months and "0" if otherwise.

My analysis also statistically controls for the proximate determinants. In this study, *age at first sexual intercourse* and *if the respondent ever had sterilization operation* are treated as proxies of the proximate determinants. These variables are controlled as proxies of the proximate determinants because the first variable indicates the respondent's biological maturation for childbearing and the second variable represents the onset of an individual's sterility. Both variable intermediate with demographic and socioeconomic factors to regulate fertility (Bongaarts, 1982; Miller & Heaton, 1991). Ideally, contraceptive use should also be controlled as a proximate determinant. In the NSFG questionnaire, however, only females are asked if they have ever used any birth control methods. For males, there is no question directly asking such information. Though men are asked their contraceptive use history associated with each of their female partners, the response rates for those questions are quite low. I thus decided not to include contraceptive use as a control variable. Age at menarche could be another proxy of the proximate determinant, indicating biological maturation for females (Miller & Heaton, 1991). Since the equivalent measure for males is not available in the NSFG dataset, this variable is not included in the analysis either.

Given that the dependent variable, CEB, is a count variable, Poisson regression is the statistical procedure used to conduct the analysis. As already noted, the Poisson model is superior to OLS or other linear models in this instance because the distribution of a count variable, such as CEB, is one that is heavily skewed with a long right tail, especially in the cases of low fertility populations. The skewed distribution of CEB could be due to the observed distribution of data having a very low mean, which reflects many women desiring few children and few women wanting many children in low fertility countries. In this case, the skewed distributions of CEB for males and for females are likely to be caused by low means of male and female CEBs.

To show the distributions of male and female CEBs, I chart the male and female CEBs in Figs. 6.1 and 6.2, respectively. In both figures, I graph the observed CEBs as compared to the predicted CEBs by estimating a univariate Poisson regression without any independent variables. Since there are no independent variables involved the univariate Poisson distribution, the univariate Poisson distribution can also be considered as a theoretical Poisson distribution in this sense. The shape of the univariate

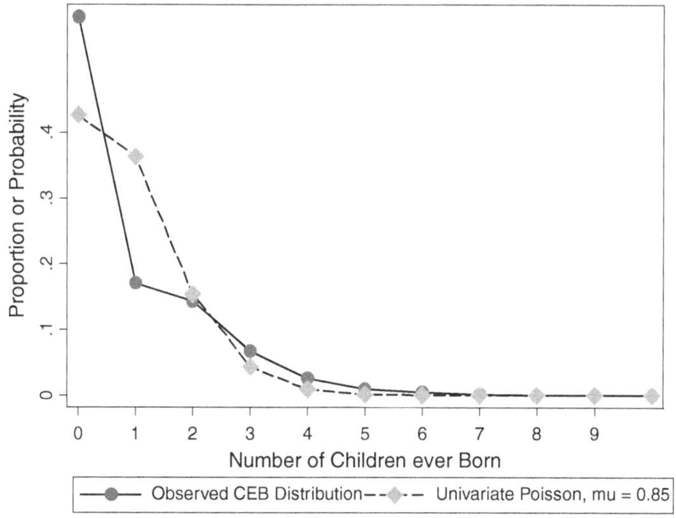

Fig. 6.1 Observed distribution and univariate poisson distribution of CEB for males with $\mu = 0.85$

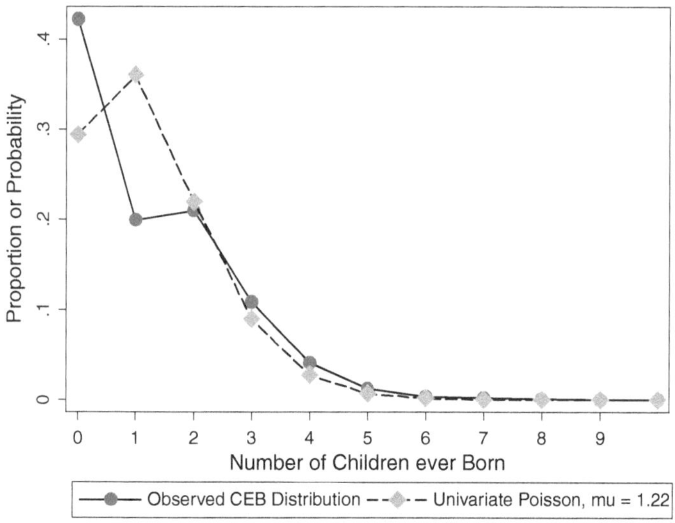

Fig. 6.2 Observed distribution and univariate poisson distribution of CEB for females with $\mu = 1.22$

Poisson distribution depends entirely on the value of the mean of the observed distribution and is based on the following formula:

$$\Pr(Y = y) = \frac{\exp(-\mu)\mu^{y}}{y!}, \quad y = 0, 1, 2, \ldots$$

Where: μ represents the mean, and y is an integer indicating number of times the count has occurred, ranging from 0 to some higher positive integer (Long & Freese, 2006). The univariate Poisson distribution aims to show the theoretical distribution of the CEB data if the data follow a Poisson distribution. In other words, what the CEB distribution would look like if the data are Poisson distributed. By contrasting the univariate Poisson distribution and the actual distribution of CEB, we can see how closely the data are Poisson distributed.

As it is shown by Fig. 6.1, the average value of CEB, μ, for males is 0.85. The Poisson theoretical/univariate distribution underpredicts men's average number of children at count zero, overpredicts counts one and two, and underpredicts counts three through six until it begins to accurately predict CEB at counts seven through nine.

Figure 6.2 displays the observed and univariate Poisson distributions of CEB for females. The average CEB for female respondents in this analysis is 1.22. The Poisson theoretical distribution underpredicts women's average number of CEB at count zero. It overpredicts counts two and three and underpredicts counts three through six. The univariate Poisson distribution is very close to the actual value of CEB at counts seven and over.

Based on these findings, I argue that despite the univariate Poisson distribution under- or over-predicts the actual values of CEB at lower counts, the distributions of CEB for both males and females are pretty much Poisson distributed. One reason for the failure of the pure Poisson distribution to perfectly fit the observed CEB data is that the numbers of children born to males or females, that is, μ, differs across the respondents. For example, the univariate Poisson distribution with a mean of 0.85 for males does not take into account the heterogeneity of the male samples in their values of μ. So it is necessary to extend the univariate Poisson distribution to the Poisson regression model, in which it is assumed that "the observed count for observation i is drawn from a Poisson distribution with mean μ, where μi, is estimated from observed characteristics," that is, from independent variables of men or women (Long & Freese, 2006, p. 356). In this case, the independent variables would be the demographic and socioeconomic variables.

The Poisson regression model is written as:

$$\mu_i = \exp\left(a + X_{1i}b_1 + X_{2i}b_2 + \ldots + X_{ki}b_k\right)$$

Where μ_i is the mean of the distribution, which is estimated from observed characteristics of the independent variables; b_i represents deviation from the mean of the omitted category, which is the reference group. The X variables are related to μ nonlinearly. In this case, μ_i is the expected number of children born to a respondent based on the respondent's demographic and socioeconomic characteristics and so forth. As compared to the univariate Poisson model, the Poisson regression model presented above includes independent variables in the model and incorporates the effects of independent variables on CEB. Since the NSFG gives different sample weights to each case, all cases in this analysis are weighted based on their final weights designated by the NSFG.

As indicated in previous chapters, the validity of male fertility reports is always a concern of researchers when studying male fertility. The problem of underreporting in the NSFG dataset has indeed been pointed out by Rendall and associates (2006) who assess fatherhood at younger ages. Considering the matter of underreporting that may have occurred in fertility reports of younger men in the NSFG dataset, my examination in this analysis is broken into two parts. The first part contains all male and female respondents and the second part includes all respondents except for males who are 25 years of age and younger. Correspondingly, the sample sizes for the two parts of analysis are 11,759 (4,117 men and 7,642 women) and 9,768 (2,126 men and 7,642 women), respectively. If differences occur when contrasting results of the two parts, then I consider the results drawn from the analysis excluding males 25 and younger as more accurate since it to a certain extent controls the bias due to underreporting of births by younger men.

6.4 Results

6.4.1 Descriptive Statistics

Table 6.1 illustrates the descriptive data for male and female respondents' fertility outcomes and their demographic and socioeconomic characteristics. According to results presented in Table 6.1, the individual fertility outcomes vary by gender. The average CEB for men is 1.2 with a standard error of 0.04. The corresponding CEB value for women is 1.3 with a standard error of 0.03. When male respondents 25 years of age or younger are eliminated from the analysis, the mean CEB for men becomes 1.5 with a standard error of 0.04. The corresponding average CEB for women aged 26 and older is 1.8 with a standard error of 0.04. These findings suggest that at the individual level, on average, males tend to have a fewer number of children than females. Nonetheless, there is a greater variation in fertility among men than among women.

A higher female than male CEB in this case may capture the reality that women on average tend to have a greater number of children than men, which echoes the finding at the aggregate level that female fertility is higher than that of males in most industrialized countries in recent years (see Chapter 2). Female CEB being higher than male CEB could also be caused by other reasons. For instance, underreporting of births by men may have led to a higher female than male fertility. This is because men are found to be more likely to omit births in fertility reports than women, especially among younger age groups and in non-marital unions. Rendall and associates (2006) has pointed out that underreporting of births does occur among younger men in the NSFG Cycle 6 dataset. Another possible explanation for a higher female than male CEB in this dataset is the age effect on fertility. As it has been pointed out, male fertility has a pattern of starting later and having a higher peak in older ages than female fertility (Paget & Timaeus, 1994). In the Cycle 6 dataset, the age range for males is from 15 to 45, which does not cover the entire reproductive span for males.

Table 6.1 Descriptive statistics for dependent, independent and control variables: U.S., 2002

	Male (all respondents)			Male (26 and over)			Female (all respondents)		
Variables	Mean (or %)	S.E.	N	Mean (or %)	S.E.	N	Mean (or %)	S. E.	N
Dependent variable									
CEB	1.2	0.04	4,117	1 5	0.04	2,126	1.3[a]	0.03	7,642
Independent variables									
Demographic factors									
Age (mean)	29.8	0.23	4,927	35.3	0.16	2,744	30.0	0.17	7,643
15–19	16.7						16.0		
20–24	16.2						16.0		
25–29	15.1						15.0		
30–34	16.6						16.7		
35–39	17.3						17.6		
40–44/45	18.2						18.7		
Race and ethnicity			4,927			2,744			7,643
Hispanic	16.7			16.2			14.8		
Non-Hispanic white	65.4			67.0			64.7		
Non-Hispanic black	11.9			10.9			14.0		
Non-Hispanic other	6.0			5.9			5.6		
Nativity-if foreign born			4,925			2,733			7,643
Native born	84.7			83.3			85.7		
Foreign born	15.3			16.7			14.3		
Metropolitan residence			4,927			2,744			7,643
MSA, central city	48.0			48.4			49.0		
MSA, other	33.3			32.4			33.3		
Not MSA	18.6			19.2			17.7		
Number of times R has been married	0.6	0.02	4,927	0.9	0.02	2,744	0.7	0.02	7,643

Table 6.1 (continued)

	Male (all respondents)			Male (26 and over)			Female (all respondents)		
Variables	Mean (or %)	S.E.	N	Mean (or %)	S.E.	N	Mean (or %)	S. E.	N
Socioeconomic factors									
Education			4,927			2,744			7,643
No diploma	22.9			15.6			21.2		
High school or less	31.5			33.5			28.3		
Some college/college	26.1			25.7			30.4		
University and above	19.5			25.3			20.1		
If R ever worked full time for 6+ months			4,925			2,742			7,636
Yes	79.1			96.7			74.1		
No	20.9			3.3			25.9		
Combined family income			4,927			2,744			7,643
Under $25,000	27.4			23.2			33.1		
$25,000–$49,999	33.3			35.4			30.3		
$50,000–$74,999	18.5			19.7			18.9		
$75,000 and over	20.8			21.8			17.7		
Proximate determinants									
Age at 1st sexual intercourse	17.0	0.08	4,108	17.4	0.1	2,612	17.3	0.06	6,785
If R ever had sterilization operation			4,925			2,742			7,643
Yes	6.4			9.8			18.2		
No	93.6			90.2			81.8		

Note: some sub-categories may not add up to 100% due to rounding.
[a]The CEB value for women who are 26 and over is 1.8 with a standard error of 0.04.
Sources: derived from NSFG Cycle 6 male and female datasets, 2002.

For the female respondents, however, the age range of 15–44 covers the reproductive years of women. Due to the gender differences in reproductive years, the age effect might be a factor that results in male CEB being relatively lower than female CEB in this dataset.

In terms of the descriptive statistics of demographic factors, male and female respondents have reported similar mean ages. There are also equivalent percentages of male and female respondents being distributed in each age group. As far as the respondent's racial and ethnic composition, the majority of the respondents reported themselves as non-Hispanic whites (65.4% for males and 64.7% for females). Hispanics and non-Hispanic Blacks count for 16.7 and 11.9% of the male respondents, and 14.8 and 14.0% of the female respondents, respectively. The rest of the 6.0% of males and 5.6% of females are other non-Hispanic racial groups, including Asians and Pacific Islanders. Thus, as compared to females, there are slightly higher percentages of Hispanic and non-Hispanic white males but a lower percentage of Non-Hispanic black males in this dataset. The percentage distributions of the male and female respondents regarding variables *nativity* and *metropolitan residence* are very similar. Overall, around 85% of the respondents reported themselves being native born. Close to 50% of the respondents lived in central cities of MSAs; one third of the respondents had their residence in other non-central city areas in MSAs, and less than 20% of the respondents lived in areas in non-MSAs. As far as the marriage variable, on average, females reported a greater average number of times being married than males (0.7 for females and 0.62 for males).

For socioeconomic indicators, a higher percentage of men (79.1%) reported that they had been in the labor force for more than 6 months as compared to women (74.1%). When combined family income is taken into consideration, descriptive results show that the U.S. women are likely to report a relatively lower family income than their male counterparts. To illustrate, around 27.0% of males reported combined family income lower than $25,000 whereas the corresponding percentage for females is 33.1%. A little over 20.0% of the male respondents reported their combined family income being higher than $75,000 in contrast to 17.7% for the female respondents. Such a gender difference shown in combined family income may be caused by the income differentials by gender and the household composition of the sampled population. Households composed by single women are likely to show a lower family income than households composed by single men since women in general have a lower average income than men. When it comes to education, there is a higher percentage of female respondents who reported having advanced educational degrees than males, particularly for the college or university graduates.

With regard to the control variables, the male and female respondents reported very similar average ages (age 17) at first sexual intercourse. However, a much higher percentage of female than male respondents (18.2% vs. 6.4%) reported having had sterilization operations. I expect that the demographic and socioeconomic factors included in the analysis influence male and female fertility outcomes through mediating with the proximate determinants. Some of these demographic and socioeconomic factors also have significantly different effects on male and female fertility.

6.4.2 Demographic Characteristics and Fertility Differentials by Gender

I now examine the effects of demographic factors on male fertility as compared to female fertility. Table 6.2 shows the association between demographic variables and childbearing, along with the gender interaction terms. As noted earlier, the gender interaction terms are generated through multiplying the gender variable by the demographic variables. The purpose of including the gender interaction terms in the models is to examine whether male fertility is impacted by the demographic/socioeconomic variables in a significantly different manner as compared to female fertility.

Model 1 focuses on the effect of age on fertility. Controlling for gender, socioeconomic factors and the proximate determinants, the Poisson regression results show that with age increasing, the average expected level of CEB increases. This effect is statistically significant, meaning that age has a significantly positive effect on CEB. The significant interaction term of age and gender shown in this model further reveals that the age effect has significantly different magnitudes on male and female fertility. Specifically, over a total range of 30 reproductive years, the expected level of CEB for women increases by 5% ($e^{0.05}$) with every 1 year increase in age. Such an age effect on male fertility is greater, that is, every 1 year increase in age raises the average expected level of CEB by 7% ($e^{0.05+0.02}$). These findings indicate a positive and greater impact of age on men's completed fertility than on women's completed fertility. These results support both hypotheses 1 and 2.

Model 2 replaces the age variable with variables representing the racial and ethnic composition of the respondent. The model shows that compared to non-Hispanic Whites, Hispanics reported the highest fertility, followed by Blacks. Other non-Hispanic racial groups do not show significantly different fertility outcomes as compared to Whites. The results show that compared to non-Hispanic Whites, having a Hispanic origin increases the respondent's expected level of CEB by 28% ($e^{0.25}$); being an African American multiplies the expected CEB level of the respondent by a factor of 1.1 ($e^{0.10}$). The interaction terms between gender and the racial and ethnic variables are not statistically significant, which suggests that men's and women's fertility outcomes are affected by their racial and ethnic composition in a similar way. These findings corroborate hypothesis 3 but challenges hypothesis 4.

In Model 3, I examine the influence of nativity on male and female fertility. Results show that foreign-born individuals tend to have a greater number of children than their native-born counterparts. Such an influence does not vary by gender, considering the interaction term of gender and nativity is not significant. My hypotheses 5 and 6 are therefore supported by empirical results.

Models 4 and 5 further investigate the effects of residence and marriage on fertility, respectively. According to previous studies, people who live in central cities of MSA should have a lower level of fertility than those who reside in other parts of MSA or non-MSA areas. Unexpectedly, the CEB of respondents who resided in non-central city areas is shown to be 10% ($e^{-0.10}$) lower than that of respondents

Table 6.2 Poisson regression of CEB on demographic factors and gender interaction terms: all male and female respondents, U.S. 2002

Variables	Model 1	Model 2	Model 3	Model 4	Model 5	Model 6
Demographic factors						
Age	0.05***					0.05***
Gender (ref. = female)	−1.03***	−0.20***	−0.16***	−0.15***	−0.39***	−0.93***
Race and ethnicity (ref. group =whites)						
Hispanic		0.25***				0.32***
Non-Hispanic black		0.10*				0.24***
Non-Hispanic other		0.10				0.18*
If foreign born (ref.= native born)			0.25***			0.04
Metropolitan residence (ref. = MSA, central city)						
MSA, other				−0.10*		−0.09
Not MSA				−0.03		0.04
Number of times R has been married					0.31***	0.18***
Gender interaction terms						
Age * male	0.02***					0.02***
Race and ethnicity (ref. group = White)						
Hispanic * male		0.03				0.14
Non-Hispanic black * male		0.12				0.07
Non-Hispanic other * male		0.22				0.21
If foreign born * male			−0.04			−0.05
Metropolitan residence (ref. = MSA, central city)						
MSA, other * male				−0.07		−0.03
Not MSA * male				0.04		−0.08
Number of times R has been married * male					0.23***	0.16**

Table 6.2 (continued)

Variables	Model 1	Model 2	Model 3	Model 4	Model 5	Model 6
Socioeconomic factors						
Highest degree R ever earned	−0.08***	−0.06***	−0.07***	−0.07***	−0.07***	−0.06***
Total combined family income	−0.01**	0.00	−0.01	−0.01	−0.01**	−0.01**
If R ever worked full time for 6+ months	0.22***	0.70***	0.71***	0.69***	0.48***	0.20**
Proximate determinants						
Age at 1st sexual intercourse	−0.02***	−0.01*	−0.01**	−0.01	−0.01	−0.02***
If R ever had sterilization operation (ref. = no)	0.36***	0.73***	0.74***	0.72***	0.52***	0.33***
Constant	−0.38***	0.25***	0.38***	0.48***	0.42***	−0.60***
N	10,877	10,877	10,850	10,877	10,877	10,850
Prob > F	0.0000	0.0000	0.0000	0.0000	0.0000	0.0000

Note: R refers to the respondent. *$p < 0.05$, **$p < 0.01$, ***$p < 0.001$ (two-tailed tests).
Sources: derived from NSFG Cycle 6 Male and Female Datasets, 2002.

who reside in central cities of MSAs. Meanwhile, the respondents in non-MSAs do not show a significantly higher fertility than respondents who resided in central cities of MSAs. The residential influence on fertility does not seem to vary by gender either, considering the non-significant gender interaction terms. These findings do not seem to corroborate hypotheses 7 and 8.

The marriage effect shown in Model 5 turns to be crucial in amplifying fertility, with a stronger impact on male than on female CEB. The significant interaction term between gender and the marriage variable suggests that on average, with every one additional marriage, men's expected CEB is multiplied by a factor of 1.71 ($e^{0.31+0.23}$); whereas for women, their expected CEB is only increased by 36% ($e^{0.23}$). These results support my hypothesis on a positive marriage effect on male and female fertility but challenge the hypothesis regarding the gender differences in the marriage and fertility relationship.

Model 6 includes all demographic characteristics, gender interaction terms and control variables in one regression model. Except for a few differences, results presented in this model are generally consistent with findings presented in separate regression models which are discussed in Models 1 through 5. The major differences of results shown in Model 6 as compared to those presented in Models 1 through 5 regard the impacts of racial and ethnic composition, nativity and marriage on childbearing. To illustrate, in the full model (Model 6), the fertility differentials caused by racial and ethnic composition increase after all demographic variables are included in the model. Meanwhile, fertility differences between non-Hispanic Whites and other non-Hispanic racial groups also become significant in model 6. Nonetheless, the influence of nativity on fertility becomes trivial. These findings suggest that after the respondent's racial and ethnic background is taken into consideration, the nativity effect on fertility disappears. Put differently, the nativity effect on fertility is likely to be caused by one's racial and ethnic background since nativity is often tangled with one's racial and ethnic composition. Such a finding eventually challenges hypothesis 5 on the nativity effect on fertility. It suggests that in the U.S., race and ethnicity may be a more important factor than nativity that determines an individual's fertility outcome. The marriage effect on fertility decreases in Model 6 as compared to Model 5. This is perhaps because the marriage effect on fertility is oppressed by some of the demographic characteristics included in the analysis.

As discussed earlier, I consider the issue of underreporting births by younger men in the analysis. Therefore, I run same regressions with male respondents 25 and younger being excluded in the models. The Poisson regression results are presented in Table 6.3. Compared to Table 6.2, results shown in Table 6.3 display a consistency with findings based on examining all respondents. The major difference lies in the coefficients of the gender variable and the gender interaction terms. The gender variable in Table 6.3 is no longer significant in the regression models. Though the gender interaction terms remain significant, the values of the interaction terms between gender and race and ethnicity become less substantial. In addition, in contrast to the stronger age effect on male than on female fertility shown in Table 6.2, age in Table 6.3 shows a stronger positive effect on female than on male fertility. On average, with every 1 year increase in age, the expected level of CEB for females is

Table 6.3 Poisson regression of CEB on demographic factors, gender interaction terms and CEB: all females and males 26 and over, U.S. 2002

Variables	Model 1	Model 2	Model 3	Model 4	Model 5	Model 6
Demographic factors						
Age	0.06***					0.05***
Gender (ref. = female)	0.34	0.01	0.07	0.07	0.02	0.34
Race and ethnicity (ref. group = White)						
Hispanic		0.21***				0.30***
Non-Hispanic black		0.09*				0.24***
Non-Hispanic other		0.08				0.18**
If foreign born (ref.= native born)			0.21***			0.02
Metropolitan residence (ref. = MSA, central city)						
MSA, other				−0.12*		−0.09*
Not MSA				−0.05		0.03
Number of times R has been married					0.33***	0.18***
Gender interaction terms						
Age * male	−0.01***					−0.02***
Race and ethnicity (ref. group = White)						
Hispanic * male		0.09				0.08
Non-Hispanic black * male		0.18*				0.05
Non-Hispanic other * male		0.22				0.18
If foreign born * male			−0.04			−0.04
Metropolitan residence (ref. = MSA, central city)						
MSA, other * male				−0.01		−0.02
Not MSA * male				0.01		−0.10
Number of times R has been married * male					0.02	0.13**

Table 6.3 (continued)

Variables	Model 1	Model 2	Model 3	Model 4	Model 5	Model 6
Socioeconomic factors						
Highest degree R ever earned	−0.08***	−0.07***	−0.07***	−0.08***	−0.07***	−0.06***
Total combined family income	−0.01**	0.00	−0.01	−0.01	−0.01**	−0.01**
If R ever worked full time for 6+ months	0.07	0.40***	0.41***	0.40***	0.25***	0.20**
Proximate determinants						
Age at 1st sexual intercourse	−0.02***	−0.01**	−0.02**	−0.01*	−0.01*	−0.02***
If R ever had sterilization operation	0.37***	0.67***	0.67***	0.65***	0.50***	0.33***
Constant	−0.35***	0.68***	0.80***	0.90***	0.68***	−0.61***
N	9,390	9,390	9,366	9,390	9,390	9,366
Prob > F	0.0000	0.0000	0.0000	0.0000	0.0000	0.0000

Note: R refers to the respondent. $^{*}p < 0.05$, $^{**}p < 0.01$, $^{***}p < 0.001$ (two-tailed tests).
Sources: derived from NSFG Cycle 6 Male and Female Datasets, 2002.

increased by 5% ($e^{0.05}$), but the CEB of males is only increased by 2% ($e^{0.05-0.02}$) (see Model 6 in Table 6.3). The inconsistency shown in both tables regarding the age effect on male and female fertility might be due to underreporting of births by younger men. As it has been documented in previous studies, younger men are more likely to underreport births than older men. Thus, when younger men are included in the analysis, age is likely to show a stronger positive effect on male than on female fertility. After younger males are eliminated from the analysis, underreporting of births by younger men is controlled to a certain extent. Then the stronger effect of age on male than on female fertility diminishes or even becomes weaker on male than on female fertility.

These findings inform us that except for the age effect, excluding younger men in the analysis does not significantly change the estimation results of how demographic characteristics influence an individual's completed fertility.

In addition to the clear effects of demographic characteristics on fertility, most control variables are found to be influential as well. The socioeconomic characteristics are treated as control variables here since this part of the analysis focuses on examining the effect of demographic variables on fertility. Education and combined family income are negatively associated with fertility outcome; employment, on the other hand, increases the respondent's fertility. As far as the proximate determinants, an earlier age at first sexual intercourse leads to a lower level of fertility; whereas the experience of having had a sterilization operation is positively related to fertility results. I will discuss these associations in later parts of this manuscript.

6.5 Socioeconomic Characteristics and Fertility Differentials by Gender

I turn now to examining the influence of socioeconomic factors on male and female fertility. Because socioeconomic status is affected by demographic characteristics, I control for demographic factors along with the proximate determinants in all models. Model 1 in Table 6.4 focuses on the effect of education on fertility with the respondents who had college degrees as the reference group. As it is shown in the model, education exhibits a negative effect on fertility. Compared to the CEB of respondents with college degrees, the expected CEB of the respondents with no diploma and with high school diploma are increased by 39% ($e^{0.33}$) and 16% ($e^{0.15}$), respectively. The expected CEB of the respondents who had university degrees is decreased by 12% ($e^{-0.13}$) compared to the reference group. The depressing effect of education on fertility reinforces hypothesis 11 on education and fertility. As regard to gender differences in the relationship of education and fertility, male and female fertility differentials appear not to be significant, considering the non-significant interaction terms between gender and the education variables. This means that education has an equivalent effect on male and female fertility, which does not support hypothesis 12 about the differential effect of education on men's and women's fertility.

Table 6.4 Poisson regression of CEB on socioeconomic factors, gender interaction terms and CEB: all male and female respondents, U.S. 2002

Variables	Model 1	Model 2	Model 3	Model 4
Socioeconomic factors				
Highest degree R ever earned (ref. = some college/college)				
No diploma	0.33***			0.28***
High school or less	0.15***			0.14***
University and above	−0.13**			−0.12**
Combined family income (ref.= $75,000 and over)				
Under $25,000		0.24***		0.13**
$25,000–$49,999		0.05		−0.03
$50,000–$74,999		−0.04		−0.06
If R ever worked full time for 6+ months (ref. = no)			−0.06	0.03
Gender interaction terms				
Highest degree R ever earned				
No diploma * male	−0.02			0.07
High school or less * male	0.05			0.05
Some college/college * male	–			–
University and above * male	0.07			0.01
Combined family income				
Under $25,000 * male		−0.16*		−0.16
$25,000–$49,999 * male		−0.02		−0.06
$50,000–$74,999 * male		0.03		−0.00
$75,000 and over * male		–		
If R ever worked full time for 6+ months * male			0.77***	0.73***

Table 6.4 (continued)

Variables	Model 1	Model 2	Model 3	Model 4
Demographic factors				
Age	0.06***	0.05***	0.05***	0.05***
Gender (ref. =female)	−0.22***	−0.12	−0.90***	−0.85***
Race and ethnicity (ref. group = White)				
Hispanic	0.39***	0.45***	0.48***	0.38***
Non-Hispanic black	0.29***	0.30***	0.34***	0.28***
Non-Hispanic other	0.30***	0.27***	0.29***	0.30***
If foreign born	0.02	0.04	0.06	0.01
Metropolitan residence (ref. = MSA, central city)				
MSA, other	−0.10*	−0.11*	−0.10*	−0.10*
Not MSA	0.03	0.05	0.08	0.02
Number of times R has been married	0.26***	0.27***	0.26***	0.26***
Proximate determinant				
Age at 1st sexual intercourse	−0.02***	−0.03***	−0.03***	−0.02***
If R ever had sterilization operation (ref.= no)	0.30***	0.32***	0.34***	0.30***
Constant	−1.59***	−1.48***	−1.20***	−1.53***
N	10,852	10,852	10,850	10,850
Prob > F	0.0000	0.0000	0.0000	0.0000

Note: R refers to the respondent. *$p < 0.05$, **$p < 0.01$, ***$p < 0.001$ (two-tailed tests).
Sources: derived from NSFG Cycle 6 male and female datasets, 2002.

In model 2 of Table 6.4, I replace the education variables with income variables. Total combined family income shows a negative effect on both male and female fertility. Such a negative effect is stronger on women's than on men's fertility. Specifically, compared to the respondents who had combined family income in 2001 over $75,000, the expected CEB for women who reported a family income lower than $25,000 is increased by 27% ($e^{0.24}$). For men, their corresponding CEB level is only increased by 8% ($e^{0.24-0.16}$). These results suggest that fertility differentials caused by combined family income is more dramatic among women than among men.

The effect of labor force participation, measured by ever working full time for more than 6 months, in model 3 shows a much stronger positive impact on male than on female fertility. On average, the CEB of men who ever worked full time for more than 6 months is twice ($e^{0.77-0.06}$) as high as the CEB of men who did not have such a working experience. For women, the effect of employment seems to be negative but not significant. These findings indicate that participating in labor force has a positive and much stronger effect on male than on female fertility. This finding has hardly been highlighted by existing demographic literature.

After I combine all socioeconomic characteristics and the gender interaction terms in model 4, the overall model suggests that the results regarding education and employment based on separate models generally persist in the combined model, with slightly decreased effects of education and employment variables on fertility (see model 4). Interestingly, the significant fertility difference by gender shown in the relationship of income and fertility in model 2 disappears in model 4. This finding suggests that controlling for other socioeconomic factors along with the gender interaction effects eliminates fertility differences by gender that are caused by income inequality. Such a finding eventually challenges hypothesis 14 on the gender differences in the fertility and income relationship.

I now replicate the statistical procedures shown in Table 6.4 but eliminate males 25 and younger. The Poisson regression results are presented in Table 6.5. Compared to findings based on analyzing all male and female respondents, significant differences occur when younger men are removed from the regression models. To illustrate, in the family income and fertility relationship, after excluding males 25 and younger, family income shows a negative effect on female fertility, but a positive effect on male fertility. That is, compared to the CEB of the respondents with over $75,000 combined family income, the expected CEB of male respondents who had family income under $25,000 is decreased by 7% ($e^{0.11-0.18}$). However, for women with the same family income, their expected CEB is increased by 12% ($e^{0.11}$). These results reveal that an increased family income leads to a higher fertility for men but a lower fertility for women. The effect of family income on male fertility turns from negative to positive after males 25 and younger are eliminated from the analysis. I am not sure how to interpret this change. There might be a combined effect between men's life cycle, income and fertility. For males who reach the age when their fertility peak occurs, family income may turn to be a factor that positively influences their fertility.

Table 6.5 Poisson regression of CEB on socioeconomic factors, gender interaction terms and CEB: all females and males 26 and Over, U.S., 2002

Variables	Model 1	Model 2	Model 3	Model 4
Socioeconomic factors				
Highest degree R ever earned (ref.=some college/college)				
No diploma	0.30***			0.28***
High school or less	0.15***			0.14***
University and above	−0.13**			−0.12**
Combined family income (ref.= $75,000 and over)				
Under $25,000		0.21***		0.11**
$25,000–$49,999		0.04		−0.03
$50,000–$74,999		−0.04		−0.06
If R ever worked full time for 6+ months (ref. = no)			−0.01	0.09
Gender interaction terms				
Highest degree R ever earned				
No diploma * male	0.02			0.07
High school or less * male	−0.01			0.01
Some college/college * male	–			–
University and above * male	−0.03			−0.06
Combined family income				
Under $25,000 * male		−0.12*		−0.18*
$25,000–$49,999 * male		−0.02		−0.08
$50,000–$74,999 * male		0.03		−0.01
$75,000 and over * male		–		
If R ever worked full time for 6+ months * male			−0.14	−0.18

Table 6.5 (continued)

Variables	Model 1	Model 2	Model 3	Model 4
Demographic factors				
Age	0.04***	0.04***	0.04***	0.04***
Gender (ref. = female)	−0.08	−0.03	0.06	0.17
Race and ethnicity (ref. group = White)				
Hispanic	0.36***	0.452***	0.45***	0.35***
Non-Hispanic black	0.28***	0.30***	0.32***	0.27***
Non-Hispanic other	0.27***	0.24***	0.25***	0.27***
If foreign born (ref. = native born)	0.02	0.04	0.06	0.02
Metropolitan residence (ref. = MSA, central city)				
MSA, other	−0.09*	−0.11*	−0.10*	−0.09*
Not MSA	0.01	0.04	0.06	0.01
Number of times R has been married	0.23***	0.25***	0.25***	0.24***
Proximate determinant				
Age at 1st sexual intercourse	−0.02***	−0.03***	−0.03***	−0.02***
If R ever had sterilization operation	0.34***	0.36***	0.37***	0.33***
Constant	−1.17***	−1.06***	−0.94***	−1.24***
N	9,368	9,368	9,366	9,366
Prob > F	0.0000	0.0000	0.0000	0.0000

Note: R refers to the respondent. $^{*}p < 0.05$, $^{**}p < 0.01$, $^{***}p < 0.001$ (two-tailed tests).
Sources: derived from NSFG Cycle 6 male and female datasets, 2002.

Another remarkable difference between results including and excluding male respondents aged 25 and younger is that the effect of labor force participation on fertility no longer varies by gender, and the main effect of labor force participation on fertility turns to be non-significant. These results undermine my hypothesis about employment and fertility. The non-significant coefficient of the employment variable is probably due to the fact that when younger men are eliminated from the analysis, the majority of the male respondents reported having had working experience, meaning there are not enough cases to make the correlation between employment and fertility significant. Another possible explanation is that the employment variable may not be a powerful measure of labor force participation. Future research needs to apply better measures to examine the fertility differentials by gender caused by an individual's employment status. Due to these reasons, my report on the effect of labor force participation and fertility will be based on the results drawn from analyzing all and female respondents.

I need to point out that in addition to the above analysis, I also ran Poisson regression that included all demographic and socioeconomic variables as well as the interaction effects between gender and demographic and socioeconomic variables (results are not shown but available from the author upon request). I find that except for the effect of racial and ethnic composition on fertility, results of including all variables are consistent with those shown in Table 6.5. The comprehensive model shows that when it comes to the racial and ethnic effect, men with Hispanic origin have an expected CEB that is 60% ($e^{0.31+0.16}$) higher than that of Caucasian men, whereas being a Hispanic woman only multiplies her expected CEB by 36% ($e^{0.31}$) as compared to being a Caucasian woman. I suspect that the fertility differentials by gender caused by racial and ethnic composition may result from the mediating effects between gender and demographic characteristics and between gender and socioeconomic factors. These effects may intertwine with each other, which makes the fertility differentials by gender significant. If it is not the case, then the results could be a statistical artifact. The conclusion and discussion part contains a more detailed discussion of this finding and its implications.

6.6 Conclusion and Discussion

This chapter has investigated the impacts of demographic and socioeconomic factors on male as compared to on female fertility. The results indicate most demographic and socioeconomic factors that are found influential on female fertility also show significant influence on male fertility. More importantly, I find that some demographic and socioeconomic variables have significantly different impacts on male and female fertility. In particular, among demographic and socioeconomic characteristics included in the analysis, age, racial and ethnic composition, marriage, labor force participation and income impact men's and women's fertility differently under certain circumstances. To specify, controlling for other factors, age significantly increases both male and female fertility, with age exhibiting a stronger effect on men's than on women's fertility when all respondents are examined. If the analysis excludes males 25 and younger, then the age effect on fertility remains positive but with a stronger positive effect on female than on male fertility. As I discussed earlier, the change in the age effect on male and female fertility after excluding younger males could be due to underreporting births by younger men. The findings therefore undermine my hypothesis on a stronger positive effect of age on male than on female fertility. However, I would like to remind the reader that since only males and female aged 15–45 are included in the analysis, this age span does not cover the entire reproductive years of men. Thus, one should interpret the research results on age and male and female fertility with caution.

As to the relationship between race and ethnicity and fertility, results show that fertility differentials resulting from racial and ethnic composition exist among both U.S. men and women. Race and ethnicity does not have significantly different impacts on men's and women's fertility until the interaction terms between gender and socioeconomic status are included in the models. This finding could be a statistical artifact because the variables and interaction terms are interrelated, one variable raises the importance of the other; or the results may have other meanings. If so, an important implication that can be drawn from the results is that the cross gender racial and ethnic effects on fertility depend on the interaction effects between gender and socioeconomic variables. Such mediating effects deserve further investigation in future research.

Marriage shows a consistently positive effect on childbearing, with a stronger impact on male than on female fertility. I expected the opposite situation to be the case, that is, marriage being more influential on female than on male fertility. To explain the discrepancy between the findings and my assumption, a causal relationship may need to be clarified first. That is, whether a stronger positive effect of marriage on male fertility indicates that marriage experience does promote men's fertility outcome to a greater extent than women's fertility; or underreporting of births in non-marital unions results in the fertility differentials by gender when marriage experience is taken into consideration. As Bachu (1996) indicates, underreporting of births happens more frequently among men than among women, especially in non-martial unions. If that is the case, then with everything else being equal, men with marriage experience tend to report a higher level of fertility than those who have no marriage experience. Though my analysis contrasts the results with and without younger men and has not found substantial differences in two sets of findings, I have not controlled the influence of omitting births in non-marital unions on fertility. Thus, whether underreporting of births by men has resulted in a stronger positive effect of marriage on male than on female fertility is worthy of further investigation. If omitting births in non-marital unions is not the reason that has caused male and female fertility differences due to marriage, then the marriage effect on distinguishing male and female fertility has an important implication. That is, an increasing number of marriages promotes men's childbearing results to a greater extent than it does on women's fertility outcome. Prior research indicates that men are more likely to remarry than women after divorce. Then findings in this research perhaps suggest that men are more likely to have births than women after divorce.

Regarding the rest of the demographic variables, my results show that nativity no longer has a significant effect on fertility once race and ethnicity is controlled. Place of residence accounts for fertility variation among the respondents, however, it does not seem to differentiate male and female fertility. These factors do not turn to be the factors that differentiate male and female fertility.

In terms of the association between socioeconomic characteristics and fertility, education shows a negative impact on fertility and its influence on fertility does not vary by gender. This is contradictory to my hypothesis since I expected education to influence men's and women's fertility in significantly different manners based on my analysis of fertility in Taiwan at the aggregate level. The occurrence of the inconsistent results perhaps indicate that in societies, such as in the U.S., where gender inequality is less of a concern, the distinguishing effect of education on male and female fertility disappears. Recall the descriptive results shown earlier that the male and female respondents reported very similar educational attainments, even with a slightly higher percentage of females reporting advanced educational degrees than males. Such equivalent percentage distributions of males and females in each educational stratum may have eradicated the differential effect of education on fertility by gender. If that is the case, then the results perhaps suggest that the differential effect of education on men's and women's fertility is likely to be caused by their unequal educational attainments. Once the educational gap by gender is closed, education is no longer a factor that distinguishes men's and women's fertility.

My review of literature in the early part of the chapter suggests that income is negatively associated with women's fertility. In this study, I use family income as a proxy and find that the income variable first served as a depressing factor of fertility, with a stronger negative effect on women's than on men's fertility. After controlling for demographic characteristics, other socioeconomic factors and the gender interaction terms, the influence of family income on fertility has changed. High family income showed a positive effect on male fertility, but a negative effect on female fertility. These results are probably caused by the fact that women with higher family income are more likely to face the role conflict between work and childbearing, which prevents them to have a greater number of children. For men, on the other hand, being in a more economically advantaged position makes them more competitive in the marriage market, and thus to produce a greater number of offspring. One may argue that in marital unions, the family income effect should not influence the husband's and the wife's fertility outcomes differently because childbearing is an ultimate decision made by both sides. As a consequence, childbearing outcomes for both the husband and the wife should be the same. This argument would be valid if the male and female respondents in the dataset were husbands and wives. In reality, however, the male and female respondents in the NSFG dataset are randomly selected samples from separate households. Thus, the argument does not weaken the validity of the research findings. I also suspect that individual income should have similar effect as family income on male and female fertility. Due to data constraint, I am not able to neither include the measure of individual income nor control other related covariates, such as costs of children, the opportunity cost of the wife's time, and other supply factors. Future research may need to take efforts to incorporate these factors in the analysis.

Regarding labor force participation and fertility, there has been a frequent emphasis on the relevance between labor force participation and women's fertility in previous literature. This research, nevertheless, shows that labor force participation in fact has a much stronger impact on men's fertility. Put differently, being in labor force substantially increases men's fertility. The mechanism behind this finding is probably similar to the one behind the association between income and men's fertility. That is, employment improves men's economic situation and therefore stimulates their fertility. The employment variable on female fertility, the reference group, is not significant in the regression models. Does this result mean that being in the labor market sector does not influence women's fertility? Researchers have pointed out that the institutional changes that occurred in recent years have eased the incompatibility between roles of mother and worker, which makes the negative association between employment and fertility nonsignificant or even turn to be positive (Rindfuss, Guzzo, & Morgan, 2003). This argument may well explain the findings of this research. Another explanation of the nonsignificant effect of the employment variable on female fertility is that the employment variable may not be the best measure of employment. Future research may consider applying better measures of employment to capture the relationship between labor force participation and female fertility.

In sum, this chapter has attempted to shed light on the mechanism of how demographic and socioeconomic factors determine men's as compared to women's fertility. The chapter has also highlighted the factors that differentiate men's and women's fertility outcomes. These factors include age, racial and ethnic composition, income, and labor force participation. It needs to be pointed out that while NSFG Cycle 6 is a rich dataset that allows detailed examination of the demographic and socioeconomic determinants of male fertility, there are still a number of limitations which cause measurement difficulties and lack of important control variables. For example, nativity is measured by place of birth, which does not take the assimilation process into consideration. In this sense, duration of residence in the U.S. could be a better measure but is not available in the dataset. While examining the effect of age on male fertility, age of the respondent's partner is not controlled. It can be an important factor because age of the respondent's partner may interact with age of the respondent and, in turn, influences male fertility. Also, the marital status of men's female partners is not controlled, which has been shown to be important in previous research (Levin & O'Hara, 1978). Future research may develop more appropriate measures and control variables to improve this current research. The most significant contributions made by this chapter are: it shows that demographic and socioeconomic covariates that are documented as influential on female fertility are found to have significant impacts on male fertility as well; age, racial and ethnic composition, income, and labor force participation are revealed to influence men's fertility in significantly different manners than women's fertility. These findings help to form fertility theories of men.

References

Alexander, K., & Reilly, T. (1981). Estimating the effects of marriage timing on educational attainment: Some procedural issues and substantive clarifications. *American Journal of Sociology, 87*, 143–156.

Anderson, J. E. (1975). The relationship between change in educational attainment and fertility rates in Taiwan. *Studies in Family Planning, 6*(3), 72–81.

Aneshensel, C. S., Fielder, E. P., & Becerra, R. M. (1989). Fertility and fertility-related behavior among Mexican American and Non-Hispanic White female adolescents. *Journal of Health and Social Behavior, 30*(1), 56–76.

Bachu, A. (1996). *Fertility of American Men*: US Census Bureau Population Division Working Paper, No.14.

Bean, F. D., Swicegood, G., & Berg, R. (2000). Mexican-origin fertility: New patterns and interpretations. *Social Science Quarterly, 81*(1), 404–420.

Ben-Porath, Y. (1973). Economic analysis of fertility in Israel: Point and counter point. *Journal of Political Economy, 81*(2), 202–233.

Bongaarts, J. (1982). The fertility-inhibiting effects of the intermediate fertility variables. *Studies in Family Planning, 13*(6), 179–189.

Borg, M. O. M. (1989). The income-fertility relationship: Effect of the net price of a child. *Demography, 26*(2), 301–310.

Budig, M. J. (2003). Are women's employment and fertility histories interdependent? An examination of causal order using event history analysis. *Social Science Research, 32*, 376–401.

Burnight, R. G., Whetten, N. L., & Waxman, B. D. (1956). Differential rural-urban fertility in Mexico. *American Sociological Review, 21*(1), 3–8.

Butz, W. P., & Ward, M. P. (1979). Will U.S. fertility remain low? A new economic interpretation. *Population and Development Review, 5*(4), 663–688.

Cameron, L. A., Dowling, M., & Worswick, C. (2001). Education and labor market participation of women in Asia: Evidence from five countries. *Economic Development and Cultural Change, 49*(3), 459–477.

Coale, A. J., & Trussell, J. (1974). Model fertility schedules: Variations in the age structure of childbearing in human populations. *Population Studies, 44*, 203–213.

Coale, A. J., & Tye, C. Y. (1961). The significance of age-patterns of fertility in high fertility populations. *The Milbank Memorial Fund Quarterly, 39*(4), 631–646.

Corijn, M., & Klijzing, E. (2001). *Transitions to adulthood in Europe*. New York, NY: Kluwer Academic Publishers.

Devaney, B. (1983). An analysis of variations in U.S. fertility and female labor force participation trends. *Demography, 20*(2), 147–161.

Dreze, J., & Murthi, M. (2001). Fertility, education, and development: Evidence from India. *Population and Development Review, 27*(1), 33–63.

Easterlin, R. A. (1973). Relative economic status and America fertility swing. In E. B. Sheldon (Ed.), *Family economic behavior* (pp. 67–90). Philadelphia, PA: J. B. Lippincott.

Forste, R., & Tienda, M. (1996). What's behind racial and ethnic fertility differentials? *Population and Development Review, 22, Supplement: Fertility in the United States: New Patterns, New Theories*, 109–133.

Freedman, D. S., & Thornto, A. (1982). Income and fertility: The elusive relationship. *Demography, 19*(1), 65–78.

Goldman, N., & Montgomery, M. (1989). Fecundability and husband's age. *Social Biology, 36*(3–4), 146–166.

Goldstein, S., & Mayer, K. B. (1965). Residence status and differences in fertility. *The Milbank Memorial Fund Quarterly, 43*(3), 291–310.

Hervitz, H. M. (1985). Selectivity, adaptation, or disruption? A comparison of alternative hypotheses on the effects of migration on fertility: The case of Brazil. *International Migration Review, 19*(2), 293–317.

Jaffe, A. J., & Cullen, R. M. (1975). Fertility of the Puerto Rican origin population-Mainland United States and Puerto Rico: 1970. *International Migration Review*, *9*(2), 193–209.

Jain, A. (1981). The effect of female education on fertility: A simple explanation. *Demography*, *18*(4), 577–595.

Johnson, N. E. (1979). Minority group status and the fertility of Black Americans. *American Journal of Sociology*, *84*, 1386–1400.

Kahn, J. R. (1994). Immigrant and native fertility during the 1980s: Adaptation and expectations for the future. *International Migration Review*, *28*(3), 501–519.

Keyfitz, N. (1977). *Applied mathematical demography*. New York, NY: Wiley.

Kravdal, O. P. (2002). Education and fertility in Sub-Saharan Africa: Individual and community effects. *Demography*, *39*(2), 233–250.

Lavely, W. R. (1986). Age patterns of Chinese marital fertility, 1950–1981. *Demography*, *23*(3), 419–434.

Lehrer, E., & Nerlove, M. (1986). Female labor force participation and fertility in the United States. *Annual Review of Sociology*, *12*, 181–204.

Levin, M. L., & O'Hara, C. J. (1978). The impact of marital history of current husband on the fertility of remarried White women in the United States. *Journal of Marriage and the Family*, *40*(1), 95–102.

Li, W. L. (1973). Temporal and spatial analysis of fertility decline in Taiwan. *Population Studies*, *27*(1), 97–104.

London, B. (1992). School-enrollment rates and trends, gender, and fertility: A cross-national analysis. *Sociology of Education*, *65*(4), 306–316.

Long, J. S., & Freese, J. (2006). *Regression models for categorical dependent variables using stata* (2nd ed.). College Station: Stata Press.

Martin, T. C. (1995). Women's education and fertility: Results from 26 demographic and health surveys. *Studies in Family Planning*, *26*(4), 187–202.

Martin, D., & Stanfors, M. A. (2006). *Education, Work and Parenthood: The Experience of Young Men and Women in Post-War Sweden*. Paper presented at the Population Association of America Annual Meetings, Los Angeles, CA.

Miller, B. C., & Heaton, T. B. (1991). Age at first sexual intercourse and the timing of marriage and childbirth. *Journal of Marriage and the Family*, *53*(3), 719–732.

Mincer, J. (1963). Market prices, opportunity costs, and income effects. In C. Crist (Ed.), *Measurement in economics*. Stanford, CA: Stanford University Press.

Mineau, G. P., & Trussell, J. (1982). A specification of marital fertility by parents' age, age at marriage and marital duration. *Demography*, *19*(3), 335–349.

Mosher, W. D., Johnson, D. P., & Horn, M. C. (1986). Religion and fertility in the United States: The importance of marriage patterns and Hispanic origin. *Demography*, *23*(3), 367–379.

Muller, E., & Cohn, R. (1977). The relation of income to fertility decisions in Taiwan. *Economic Development and Cultural Change*, *25*(2), 325–347.

National Center for Health Statistics (2005). *Fertility, family planning and reproductive health of U.S. women: Data from the 2002 national survey of family growth*. Maryland, MD: Hyattsville.

Okore, A. O. (1980). Rural-urban fertility differentials in Southern Nigeria: An assessment of some available evidence. *Population Studies*, *34*(1), 171–179.

Paget, W. J., & Timaeus, I. M. (1994). A relational Gompertz model of male fertility: Development and assessment. *Population Studies*, *48*(2), 333–340.

Poston, J., & Dudley, L. (2000). Social and economic development and the fertility transitions in Mainland China and Taiwan. *Population and Development Review*, *26*, *Supplement*, 40–60.

Rendall, M. S., Joyner, K., Peters, H. E., Yang, F., Handcock, M. S., & Ryan, A. (2006). *A Bayesian Approach to Combining Population and Survey Data for Male Fertility Estimation*. Paper presented at the Annual Meetings of Population Association of America, Los Angeles, CA.

Rindfuss, R. R., Bumpass, L., & John, C. S. (1980). Education and fertility: Implications for the role women occupy. *American Sociological Review*, *45*(3), 431–447.

Rindfuss, R. R., Guzzo, K. B., & Morgan, S. P. (2003). The changing institutional context f low fertility. *Population Research and Policy Review*, *21*(5–6), 411–438.
Rindfuss, R. R., Morgan, P., & Offutt, K. (1996). Education and the changing age pattern of American fertility: 1963–1989. *Demography*, *33*(3), 277–290.
Robinson, W. C. (1963). Urbanization and fertility: The Non-Western experience. *The Milbank Memorial Fund Quarterly*, *41*(3), 291–308.
Rodrigues, G., & Cleland, J. (1981). The effects of socioeconomic characteristics on fertility in 20 countries. *International Family Planning Perspectives*, *7*(3), 93–101.
Saenz, R. (2004). *Latinos and the Changing Face of American at the Turn of the Century*: Population Reference Bureau, Russell Sage Foundation Census 2000 Publication Series.
Saenz, R., & Morales, M. C. (2005). Demography of race and ethnicity. In J. Poston, L. Dudley, & M. Micklin (Eds.), *Handbook of population*. New York, NY: Academics/Klewers.
Sanchez, J. J. (1998). Relationships between nuptiality and fertility: A case study on the Spanish province of Navarre, 1786–1991. *Population Studies*, *52*(1), 105–115.
Singley, S. G., & Landale, N. S. (1998). Incorporating origin and process in migration fertility frameworks: The case of Puerto Rican women. *Social Forces*, *76*(4), 1437–1464.
Skirbekk, V., Kohler, H. -P., & Prskawetz, A. (2004). Birth month, school graduation, and the timing of births and marriages. *Demography*, *41*(3), 547–568.
Smith-Lovin, L., & Tickamyer, A. R. (1978). Nonrecursive models of labor force participation, fertility behavior and sex role attitudes. *American Sociological Review*, *43*(4), 541–557.
South, S. J., & Baumer, E. P. (2000). Deciphering community and race effects on adolescent premarital childbearing. *Social Forces*, *78*(4), 1379–1408.
Stephen, E. H., & Bean, F. D. (1992). Assimilation, disruption and the fertility of Mexican-origin women in the United States. *International Migration Review*, *26*(1), 67–88.
Teachman, J. D., & Polonko, K. A. (1988). Marriage, parenthood, and the college enrollment of men and women. *Social Forces*, *67*(2), 512–523.
Thornto, A. (1978). The relationship between fertility and income, relative income, and expected well-being. In J. Simon (Ed.), *Research in population economics* (Vol. I), Greenwich, CT: JAI Press.
van de Walle, F. (1980). Education and the demographic transition in Switzerland. *Population and Development Review*, *6*(3), 463–472.
Waite, L. J., & Stolzenberg, R. M. (1976). Intended childbearing and labor force participation of young women: Insights from nonrecursive models. *American Sociological Review*, *41*(2), 235–251.
Watkins, S. (1986). Conclusions. In A. J. Coale & S. Watkins (Eds.), *The decline of fertility in Europe*. Princeton, NJ: Princeton University Press.
Weinberger, M. B. (1987). The relationship between women's education and fertility: Selected findings from the world fertility surveys. *International Family Planning Perspectives*, *13*(2), 35–46.
Westoff, C., & Ryder, N. (1977). *The contraceptive revolution*. Princeton, NJ: Princeton University Press.
Wildsmith, E., & Raley, R. K. (May 2006). Race-ethnic differences in nonmarital fertility: A focus on Mexican American women. *Journal of Marriage and Family*, *68*, 491–508.
Wood, J. W., & Weinstein, M. (1988). A model of age-specific fecundability. *Population Studies*, *42*, 85–113.
Xie, Y., & Pimentel, E. E. (1992). Age patterns of marital fertility: Revising the Coale-Trussell method. *Journal of the American Statistical Association*, *87*(420), 977–984.
Zeng, Y., & Vaupel, J. W. (1989). The impact of urbanization and delayed childbearing on population growth and aging in China. *Population and Development Review*, *15*(3), 425–445.
Zeng, Y., Vaupel, J. W., & Yashin, A. I. (1985). Marriage and fertility in China: A graphical analysis. *Population and Development Review*, *11*(4), 721–736.

Chapter 7
Religion, Religiosity and Male and Female Fertility

Similar to the vast interest in examining how demographic and socioeconomic factors determine fertility, demographers and sociologists over many decades have documented fertility differentials across religious groups. Most studies of religion and fertility in the United States elaborate female fertility differentials among people who are affiliated with various religious denominations (Janssen & Hauser, 1981; Lehrer, 1996, 2004; Marcum, 1988; Mosher, Johnson, & Horn, 1986; Poston, 1990). Catholic women often are reported as having a particularly high level of fertility. Protestant women's fertility is shown to be lower than that of Catholics and is located in the middle of the continuum. Non-Orthodox Jews are at the end of the continuum and have consistently shown the lowest fertility rate among all religious groups in the U.S. (Lehrer, 2004; Sander, 1993). In recent years, however, demographers have reported that fertility differences among Catholics and other religious groups have been shrinking, and that Protestants' fertility tends to be higher than that of Catholics and other religious groups (Mosher et al., 1986; National Center for Health Statistics, 2005; Westoff & Jone, 1979). In this chapter, I will focus the examination on contrasting men's and women's fertility differentials across various religious denominations. In addition, I consider the effect of religiosity on fertility. I investigate whether for both males and females who are more engaged in religion, they tend to have a greater number of children regardless of their religious denominations. For instance, fundamentalist Protestant religious doctrines are pronatalist, which forbid artificial forms of contraception, resist abortion, and favor relatively larger families (Lehrer, 1996; Marcum, 1981). Meanwhile, on average, fundamentalist Protestants also have a stronger religiosity compared to other religious groups: they attend religious services more frequently than people of other religious denominations (Lehrer, 2004). Previous literature rarely examines whether the higher fertility rate of fundamentalist Protestants is caused by their greater level of religiosity by attending church services more often or is caused by the religious teaching of their denomination regarding favoring more children. In this chapter, I intend to fill the gaps of previous analyses by empirically examining: (1) how religious affiliation and religiosity affect men's fertility; (2) whether men's and women's fertility outcomes are impacted by religious affiliation and religiosity in significantly different manners. I will set forth a series of hypotheses to examine

L. Zhang, *Male Fertility Patterns and Determinants*, The Springer Series on Demographic Methods and Population Analysis 27, DOI 10.1007/978-90-481-8939-7_7,

these issues in this chapter, followed by empirical tests of the hypotheses. Before I do so, I will first review several major theories that explain fertility differentials across religious groups.

7.1 Theories on Religion and Fertility

Four principal theories have been proposed in the literature of fertility to explain fertility differentials across religious groups, namely, (1) the particularized theology hypothesis, (2) the characteristics hypothesis, (3) the minority status hypothesis, and (4) the social interaction hypothesis (Chamie, 1981; McQuillan, 2004). The particularized theology theory views fertility differentials as a result of specific doctrinal differences among religions. According to this perspective, religious groups whose doctrines are against contraception and abortion and favor a large family size should have a higher fertility rate. For those religious groups who do not have such doctrines, the fertility rate should be lower. Examples of religious groups with these doctrines include Roman Catholics, fundamentalist Protestants, Latter-Day Saints (Mormons), and Amish. Religious groups who have no proscriptions on birth control are, for example, mainstream Protestants and Jews (Jurecki-Tiller, 2004). Empirical research has provided some evidence for the particularized theology hypothesis by demonstrating that mainstream Protestants and Jews have higher levels of contraceptive use and lower fertility rates as compared to Catholics and fundamentalist Protestants (De Jong, 1965; Freedman, Whelpton, & Smith, 1961; Mosher & Hendershot, 1984; Mosher, Williams, & Johnson, 1992).

The characteristics theory argues that the fertility differentials among religious groups are not caused by religious doctrines. Rather, demographic and socioeconomic differentials of the members of religious groups result in their fertility differences. Once demographic and socioeconomic statuses of religious groups are controlled, fertility differentials among religious groups should disappear. The characteristics hypothesis also is supported by previous findings. For instance, the U.S. Catholic and non-Catholic fertility differentials disappear after controlling for their members' socioeconomic status (Westoff & Jone, 1979). Muslim fertility is found to be largely impacted by differences in socioeconomic conditions as well (Johnson-Hanks, 2006).

The third perspective, the minority group status theory, contends that the insecurity of minority group status plays a role in depressing fertility of minority religious groups below that of the majority. The prerequisites for the minority status mechanism to operate are: (1) acculturation; (2) socioeconomic mobility; and (3) no pronatalist ideology or norms (Goldscheider, 1971, p. 297). This approach is not only used to explain fertility differentials among religious groups, but is also used to account for fertility differentials among racial and ethnic groups (Poston, Chang, & Dan, 2006). The definition of minority group status according to this approach is based on the numerical size of the group and whether a racial and ethnic group is considered psychologically as a minority. Examples of such groups are South

African blacks and Latinos. In some parts of the U.S., these two groups may be a numerical majority but are still psychologically treated as minorities (Bouvier & Rao, 1975; Chamie, 1981). Part of the empirical support of this perspective comes from the low fertility level of Jews, which often is believed to be associated with their minority status (Goldscheider & Uhlenberg, 1969; Lehrer, 2004).

The last theory, the interaction approach, also is referred to as the socialization hypothesis. This hypothesis highlights the role of social interaction in shaping reproductive behavior (Bongaarts & Watkins, 1996; Montgomery & Casterline, 1996; Watkins, 1992). It believes that religious institutions are a major source of social exposure through which members of a certain religious group adopt their religious doctrines and are impacted by other members' fertility behavior. Such an approach is in line with the social networks theory and the "diffusion theory" of fertility which emphasize the role of interaction in shaping behavior and the diffusion effect of family planning ideology in influencing fertility (Coale & Watkins, 1986; Watkins, 1992). Such a perspective also echoes the idea that "fertility is an aggregate property, a characteristic of the groups to which the couple belong and not directly of the couple themselves" (Ryder, 1974, p. 76). Recent research shows more and more support for this hypothesis (Knodel, Gray, Sriwatchrin, & Peracca, 1999; Marchena & Waite, 2001; Ongaro, 2001; Yeatman & Trinitapoli, 2007).

Previous studies of religion and fertility along with the four theoretical approaches have increased considerably our understanding of the relationship between religion and fertility. However, these studies and approaches mainly have focused on female fertility. The way in which male fertility is impacted by religion largely has been ignored. Meanwhile, as noted earlier, these studies have emphasized primarily fertility differentials among people who belong to various religious denominations. The effect of religiosity on fertility appears to have eluded researchers. In the following sub-sections of the chapter, I will incorporate male fertility and religiosity into the analysis of fertility and religion. Below, I set forth a series of hypotheses to examine these subject matters.

7.2 Research Hypotheses

I now present my hypotheses regarding the subject matters of this research. My first a few hypotheses regard the impact of religiosity on male and female fertility. Religiosity is an important aspect of religion which often is viewed as the intensity of religious beliefs and participation (Myers, 1996). Religious beliefs are, notably, beliefs in hell, heaven, and an afterlife. Religious participation includes such behaviors as church attendance, participating in church-related activities, viewing/listening to religious broadcasts, and reading the holy books of the religion (Barro & McCleary, 2003; Corijn, 2001; Myers, 1996). Strong religiosity usually is marked by strong daily influence of religious beliefs on individual decisions and frequent participation in religious activities.

Although previous religious studies mainly focus on examining fertility differences among religious groups, empirical analyses have shown some evidence that religiosity impacts demographic behavior. In terms of the effect of religious participation on fertility and fertility-related behavior, researchers observe that religious participation among young people is linked strongly to more positive attitudes towards marriage and having children (Marchena & Waite, 2001). Analyzing the 1985 and 1999 Spanish fertility Surveys, Adsera (2007) shows that in Spain, church participation plays an important role in shaping people's fertility behavior. Individuals who seldom participate in church activities are found tend to delay significantly their timing of first parenthood, controlling for all other factors (Ongaro, 2001).

Then why does religious participation influence people's demographic behavior? The social networks approach and the "diffusion theory" of fertility may provide explanations for this mechanism. According to the social networks perspective, religious people build their social networks by attending church activities. Regular churchgoers are connected more strongly to their religious groups, that is, their social networks. As a consequence, they are more likely to accept the religious doctrines of their churches. In terms of their reproductive behavior, regular church goers are thus more likely to be influenced by their church teachings of childbearing as well as by the patterns of other church members' fertility behavior. In a similar vein, the "diffusion theory," initiated by Princeton demographers, explains the effect of religious participation by looking at the role of cultural diffusion and social interaction in spreading new cultural models of reproduction, that is, birth control and family planning (Coale & Watkins, 1986; Watkins, 1992). For those who participate religious activities more frequently, they should be more likely to be influenced by their religious doctrines and less likely to be influenced by other cultural norms. Based on the empirical findings and these explanations, I expect church participation to be highly influential on both male and female fertility. So my first hypothesis is as follows:

Hypothesis 1: The more frequently people attend religious services, the more children they will have, controlling for religious affiliation and other factors.

Besides religious participation, religious beliefs also are important. In Austria, researchers observe that non-religious persons have a lower marital rate than religious persons. Non-religious women also have a lower rate of having first birth than their religious counterparts (Preiffer & Nowak, 2001). A similar pattern also is found in other European countries such as Britain and Italy (Berrington, 2001; Ongaro, 2001). Additionally, Westoff and Frejka (2007) examine fertility patterns among European Muslim women and find that fertility is directly correlated with their religious beliefs. Muslim women have a significantly higher level of fertility than non-Muslim women who are less religious and hold less strong family values. If "no religion" is considered as one extreme on the religiosity scale, then empirical findings seem to suggest that being more religious or having stronger religious beliefs is related positively to early marriage and a higher likelihood of giving first birth in early ages. Such a positive effect can be explained by the fact that most religions encourage marriage and highly value the family. Since the majority of fertility behavior does occur within marital unions in most countries (Bongaarts, 1982; Hervitz, 1985; Mosher et al., 1986), having stronger religious beliefs is expected to have a positive effect on fertility. Based on this rationale and findings of previous research, I predict strong religious beliefs to have a positive effect on fertility, controlling for religious affiliation and other factors. Such a positive association works on both men's and women's fertility. So my hypothesis on religiosity and fertility is set forth as follows:

Hypothesis 2: People who have strong religious beliefs are more likely to have a greater number of children than people without such beliefs, controlling for religious affiliation and other factors.

Since I am also interested in investigating whether religiosity has significantly different effects on male and female fertility, I propose research hypotheses on the gender differences in the religiosity and fertility relationship. The hypotheses of my research are based on findings of previous analyses. Previous studies have suggested that, in general, women's fertility behavior is more likely to be impacted by religious values and beliefs as compared to men (Corijn & Klijzing, 2001; Goldscheider & Goldscheider, 1993). One research conducted by Preiffer and Nowak's (2001), however, shows that in Austria, men are more likely to be influenced by religion in terms of marriage and childbearing. Berrington (2001) further shows that in Britain, people with stronger levels of religiosity are more likely to marry early and give birth to children, but such a pattern does not differ among men and women. Due to the fact that the majority of prior studies support a stronger influence of religiosity on female than on male fertility, my hypotheses are thus set as follows:

Hypothesis 3: Religious participation promotes women's fertility to a greater extent than men's fertility, controlling for other factors. And,

Hypothesis 4: Religious beliefs have a stronger push effect on women's fertility than on men's, controlling for other factors.

As far as the fertility differentials across religious groups, though abundant of literature has highlighted fertility differences among women with various religious denominations, previous research has rarely taken men and their fertility into consideration. Despite a few studies have contrasted the religious impacts on men's and women's fertility and fertility related behavior, there is hardly any evidence that demonstrates gender differences in the correlation between fertility and religious affiliation. For instance, Janssen and Hauser (1981) have examined the effects of religious and secular socialization on Wisconsin men's and women's fertility. Their findings confirm a positive relationship between Catholic religion and the preference for having more children without showing significant gender differentials. Thus, in this research, I propose the following hypotheses for testing:

Hypothesis 5: The fertility differentials are shown among both males and females with various religious denominations, controlling for other factors. And,

Hypothesis 6: There are no significant gender differences regarding fertility differentials among religious groups, controlling for other factors.

Because I hypothesize that religiosity has a positive effect on fertility, I predict that fertility differentials among various religious groups may be due partly to the level of religiosity among members of religious groups. Thus, I propose the following hypotheses and I expect there is no significant gender difference:

Hypothesis 7: Fertility differentials among various religious groups will decrease once religiosity is taken into consideration, controlling for other factors. And,

Hypothesis 8: The mediating effect of religiosity on fertility through religious denomination does not vary by gender.

The above hypotheses will be statistically tested in the following sub-sections. I now move to the introduction of data, variables and methods that are applied in the analysis.

7.3 Data, Methods and Variables

So far, I have formulated hypotheses on the impacts of religion and religiosity on male fertility as compared to female fertility. Next, I will move to the empirical analysis that tests these hypotheses. For the tests of my hypotheses, I use data from the 2002 NSFG Cycle 6 to conduct the analysis. As already noted in previous chapter, the NSFG Cycle 6 dataset contains rich information on fertility, marriage, cohabitation, contraception, and related issues. Meanwhile, the Cycle 6 survey also included measures of religious affiliation, religious attendance and religious beliefs. Also included are usual demographic and socioeconomic characteristics of the respondent. In all, 4,928 men and 7,643 women were interviewed in the survey. Similar to Chapter 6, I combine the female and male datasets together for the purpose of generating gender interaction terms in order to test whether the impacts of religion and religiosity on fertility vary by gender.

The dependent variable used in the research is fertility, which is again measured by the number of children ever born (CEB) to a male or a female respondent. Given that CEB is a count variable, I apply Poisson regression as the statistical model to conduct the analysis.

The main independent variables are the religious variables, namely, religious affiliation and religiosity. The religious affiliation variable is operationalized as the respondent's current religious domination, which is classified as a set of four dummy variables: Catholic, fundamentalist Protestant, other Protestant, and other non-Christian religion. This classification follows that of the 2002 NSFG reports (National Center for Health Statistics, 2005). Among those, fundamentalist Protestants include Baptists/Southern Baptists; other Protestants include Methodists, Lutherans, Presbyterians and Episcopalians.

Religiosity is measured by two variables, which are *frequency the respondent attends religious services* and *the importance of religion in the respondent's daily life*. These measurements capture the behavior and belief dimensions of religiosity, respectively. Since there is no question directly asking the strength of religious belief in the NSFG questionnaire, *the importance of religion in the respondent's daily life* is used as the question measuring the strength of religious beliefs. For people who are affiliated with certain religious dominations, possible responses for the religious participation variable are: more than once a week, once a week, 1–3 times per month, and less than once a month. Responses for the religious beliefs item are: very important, somewhat important, and not important. Note that the religious belief measurement in the NSFG dataset is inapplicable for those respondents who claim themselves having no religious affiliations. The data restriction allows me to only include respondents who claimed to be affiliated with religious denominations to examine the effect of religiosity on fertility. As such, 3,247 men and 6,513 women are analyzed in the regression models. In order to provide information of the respondents who are eliminated from the analysis, I present some demographic and socioeconomic characteristics of those people in Table 7.2.

The NSFG questionnaire does contain questions associated with the respondents' religious denomination and religiosity during their upbringing, which measure religious affiliation and the frequency of religious service attendance at age 14. But my preliminary analysis does not show significant effects of these variables on CEB. Thus, I decided not to use those variables in the analysis.

My analysis also controls for some established covariates that influence fertility. These include demographic factors such as age, race and ethnicity, nativity, and marital status (Coale & Trussell, 1974; Jaffe & Cullen, 1975; Saenz & Morales, 2005; Singley & Landale, 1998; Xie & Pimentel, 1992), and socioeconomic factors, for example, educational attainment, employment status, and income (Ballard, 2004; Ellison, Echevarria, & Smith, 2005; Lehrer, 1996; Sander, 1992). These variables are used as control variables in the equations predicting both male and female fertility. Gender is also controlled in the combined dataset.

In terms of the measurement of these control variables, age is measured in years. Respondent's race and ethnicity is measured via categorizing the respondent into one of the following four racial and ethnic groups: Hispanic origin, non-Hispanic White, Black, and other. Marital status is set as a dummy variable which is coded as "1" if ever married and "0" if otherwise. Nativity is a dummy variable coded as "1" if the respondent is foreign born and "0" if otherwise. The variable gender is coded as "1" if male and "0" if female. Females are treated as the reference group. I use the highest degree received to represent the respondent's educational attainment. For employment status, I code it as "1" if the respondent ever worked and "0" if otherwise. Income is measured by total combined gross family income in 2001, which is coded into four categories, ranging from under $25,000 to $75,000 or more.

7.4 Results

7.4.1 Descriptive Results

Basic descriptive statistics of variables are displayed in Tables 7.1 and 7.2. Note all of the information presented in Table 7.1 is only for people who claimed themselves being affiliated with certain religions. Information for non-religious respondents is presented in Table 7.2. Sample weights are applied to the descriptive analysis of each variable.

Results show that women tend to report a higher level of CEB than men for both religious and non-religious people. The mean CEB for all females and females 26 and over are 1.3 and 1.8, with a standard error of 0.04 and 0.03, respectively. The corresponding values for all males and male respondents 26 and over are 1.2 with a standard deviation of 0.05 and 1.5 with a standard error of 0.05, respectively. These figures indicate that at the individual level, men on average have a fewer number of children than women. However, there is more variation in fertility outcome among men than among women.

When the CEBs of religious and non-religious groups are compared, it is clear that religious people tend to have a greater number of children than their non-religious counterparts. For men, the average CEB for the religious group is 1.2, whereas the corresponding value for the non-religious group is 0.8. Religious women reported an average CEB of 1.3 as compared to the average CEB of 1.0 reported by non-religious women. In addition, fertility of non-religious males tend to show more variation than that of their female counterparts for religious and non-religious groups.

In terms of the independent variables, Catholicism seems to be the most popular religion for all male respondents who claimed religion affiliations (35.4%), followed by other Protestant religions (31%), fundamentalist Protestant religions (24.1%), and other non-Christian religions (9.5%). When only males who are 26 and over are considered, respondents who are affiliated with other Protestant religions (34.9%) and fundamentalist Protestant (31.2%) surpass those who claimed themselves as Catholics (24.1%). More young men are affiliated with Catholic religion than other religious affiliations is probably because although there has been a decline across cohorts in the propensity to declare religious beliefs, Catholic males are to a certain extent "immune" to this decline. For females, there are higher percentages of the respondents who claimed themselves as fundamentalist Protestants or other Protestants. The descriptive results seem to suggest that compared to all male respondents, the distribution pattern of male respondents who are 26 and over in various religious denominations is more similar to that of the female respondents.

As far as religious participation is concerned, all male respondents and those who are 26 and older do not show significantly different patterns. The majority (around 30%) of the two sets of men reported attending religious services less than once a month, whereas female respondents show a pattern of attending religious services more frequently than males. In general, there are higher percentages of females who

Table 7.1 Descriptive statistics for respondents who claimed religious affiliations: U.S., 2002

Variables	Male (all respondents)			Male (26 and over)			Female (all respondents)		
	Mean (or %)	SD	N	Mean (or %)	SD	N	Mean (or %)	SD	N
Dependent variable									
CEB	1.2	0.05	3, 247	1.5	0.05	2, 126	1.3[a]	0.03	6, 512
Independent variables									
Religious affiliation			3, 938			2, 222			6, 513
Catholic	35.4			24.1			26.8		
Fundamentalist Protestant	24.1			31.2			33.0		
Other Protestant	31.0			34.9			33.4		
Other non-Christian	9.5			9.8			6.9		
Frequency of attending religious services			3, 938			2, 219			6, 507
More than once a week	10.7			10.0			14.1		
Once a week	23.0			23.1			25.3		
1–3 times per month	19.0			18.9			19.2		
Less than once a month	29.0			30.2			28.0		
Never	18.4			17.8			13.4		
Importance of religious beliefs			3, 920			2, 215			6, 495
Very important	47.5			49.5			57.9		
Some important	40.3			38.3			36.1		
Not important	12.2			12.2			6.0		
Control variables									
Demographic factors									
Age	29.9	0.24	3, 938	35.3	0.19	2, 222	30.1	0.19	6, 513
Race and ethnicity			3, 938			2, 222			6, 513
Hispanic	17.8			17.5			15.3		
Non-Hispanic white	63.4			64.6			64.5		
Non-Hispanic black	12.5			11.5			14.7		
Non-Hispanic other	6.3			6.5			5.5		

Table 7.1 (continued)

Variables	Male (all respondents)			Male (26 and over)			Female (all respondents)		
	Mean (or %)	SD	N	Mean (or %)	SD	N	Mean (or %)	SD	N
Nativity-if foreign born			3,938			2,222			6,499
Native born	96.1			84.0			85.5		
Foreign born	4.0			16.0			14.5		
If R ever married			3,938			2,222			6,513
Yes	46.7			75.6			59.5		
No	53.3			24.4			40.5		
Socioeconomic factors									
Education			3,938			2,222			6,513
No diploma	22.6			22.7			21.1		
High school or less	31.6			31.6			27.6		
Some college/college	26.9			26.8			29.2		
University and above	18.9			19.0			22.2		
If R ever worked			3,938			2,222			6,513
Yes	95.0			99.0			90.1		
No	5.0			1.0			9.9		
Combined family income			3,938			2,222			6,513
$24,999 and under	29.4			24.7			32.8		
$25,000–$49,999	33.3			35.1			30.4		
$50,000–$74,999	18.3			19.6			19.1		
$75,000 and above	20.8			21.6			17.7		

[a]The CEB for women 26 and over is 1.8 with a standard error of 0.04.
Sources: derived from NSFG Cycle 6 male and female datasets, 2002.

Table 7.2 Descriptive statistics for respondents who did not claim religious affiliations: U.S., 2002

Variables	Male (all respondents)			Male (26 and over)			Female (all respondents)		
	Mean (or %)	SD	N	Mean (or %)	SD	N	Mean (or %)	SD	N
Dependent variable									
CEB	0.82	0.05	856	1.15	0.05	487	1.03[a]	0.03	1,107
Independent variables			–			–			–
Religious affiliation	–			–			–		
Frequency of attending religious services	–			–			–		
Importance of religious beliefs	–			–			–		
Control variables									
Demographic factors									
Age	29.3	0.24	972	35.3	0.19	512	29.0	0.20	1,107
Race and ethnicity			972			512			1,107
Hispanic	12.0			10.0			11.7		
Non-Hispanic white	74.0			78.6			73.2		
Non-Hispanic black	9.3			8.3			9.3		
Non-Hispanic other	4.8			3.1			5.8		
Nativity-if foreign born			971			511			1,109
Native born	87.4			87.9			86.9		
Foreign born	12.6			12.1			13.1		
If R ever married			3,938			512			1,107
Yes	39.2			60.6			50.0		
No	60.8			39.4			50.0		
Socioeconomic factors									
Education			972			512			1,107
No diploma	24.4			16.0			22.2		
High school or less	30.9			32.7			30.5		
Some college/college	22.5			19.2			26.3		
University and above	22.2			32.1			21.0		

Table 7.2 (continued)

Variables	Male (all respondents)			Male (26 and over)			Female (all respondents)		
	Mean (or %)	SD	N	Mean (or %)	SD	N	Mean (or %)	SD	N
If R ever worked			972			512			1, 107
Yes	93.3			99.1			91.6		
No	6.7			0.9			8.4		
Combined family income			972			512			1, 107
$24,999 and under	34.3			19.8			34.9		
$25,000–$49,999	33.1			37.0			28.9		
$50,000–$74,999	11.9			21.1			17.8		
$75,000 and above	20.7			22.1			18.4		

Note: some sub-categories may not add up to 100% due to rounding.
[a]The CEB value for women who are 26 and over is 1.43 with a standard error of 0.04.
Sources: derived from NSFG Cycle 6 male and female datasets, 2002.

reported attending religious services frequently than males. For instance, around 14% of females reported that they attended religious services more than once a week; the corresponding percentage for males is 10.7%. Also, 25.3% of females and 23.0% of males reported that they attended religious services once a week, respectively.

Compared to males, females also tend to consider religious beliefs to be important. For instance, around 58% of the female respondents considered religious beliefs as "very important" in their daily lives, compared to 49.5% of the male respondents 26 and over, and 47.5% of all male respondents. These results indicate that women are more likely to have a higher level of religiosity which is measured by religious beliefs as compared to men; and older men tend to be more engaged in religion as compared to younger men.

Regarding the demographic characteristics of all respondents, there is a higher percentage of Hispanic males than females and a lower percentage of black males than females in the dataset. The percentage of married women is higher than that of married men, which could be another reason for a higher female than male fertility rate. In terms of the socioeconomic characteristics, men 26 and over reported a higher total combined family income as compared to the sub-groups that include all male and female respondents. In general, men tend to report a higher total combined family income than women. The percentage of men who ever participated in the labor force is also higher than that of women, 99.0% vs. 90.1%. As already indicated in Chapter 6, a higher percentage of female respondents reported having advanced educational degrees as compared to their male counterparts.

When the religious and non-religious groups are compared, the average age of non-religious respondents is similar to that of their religious counterparts. If race and ethnicity are taken into consideration, then non-religious respondents tend to be composed by a higher percentage of non-Hispanic whites and lower percentages of other racial and ethnic groups. In this sense, other racial and ethnic groups other than non-Hispanic whites tend to be more religious than non-Hispanic whites. Moreover, non-religious male respondents are likely to be composed by a higher percentage of foreign born population, whereas a reverse pattern is shown among female respondents and male respondents who are 26 and over. In addition, non-religious population is more likely to stay single than religious population. Some differences are also shown when the socioeconomic characteristics of the religious and non-religious groups are compared. Specifically, there is a higher percentage of men with advanced degrees among non-religious than religious respondents. For women, an opposite situation seems to be true, that is, a higher percentage of non-religious women reported high school or lower educational attainments as compared to their religious counterparts. These findings suggest a gender difference in educational attainments associated with religion. That is, having no religious affiliation is likely to be associated with a higher educational attainment for men but a lower educational attainment for women. Only marginal differences are shown with regard to employment status among non-religious and religious population. For family income, compared to religious respondents, higher percentages of non-religious female respondents and male respondents 26 and over are distributed to higher family income categories (categories with family income above $50,000). Put differently, the non-religious group seems to be in a more economically advantaged position than the religious group if family income is used as an indicator.

These demographic and socioeconomic differentiations between religious and non-religious groups suggest that it is necessary to examine fertility differences due to demographic and socioeconomic differentials among religious and non-religious groups. Due to data constraint, I am not able to include the non-religious group in this analysis. Future research may extend the analysis to comparing fertility of religious and non-religious groups.

7.4.2 Statistical Methods and Results

Given that CEB is a count variable, Poisson regression is the statistical procedure used to conduct the analysis. The Poisson regression can be expressed by the following model:

$$\mu_i = \exp(a + X_{1i}b_1 + X_{2i}b_2 + \cdots X_{ki}b_k)$$

Where μ_i is the mean of the distribution, which is estimated from observed characteristics of the independent variables; a is the constant; b_i represents deviation from the mean of the omitted category, which is the reference group. The X variables are related to μ nonlinearly. In this case, μ_i is the expected number of children born to a respondent based on the respondent's religious affiliation, level of religiosity, and so forth. All cases are weighted based on the final weights of each sample given by the NSFG.

Table 7.3 presents the Poisson regression results analyzing the combined dataset with all male and female respondents. In model 1, I include the religious affiliation variable and socioeconomic characteristics as the control variables. As it can be seen, compared to being Catholics, being members of other non-Christian religions multiplies the expected number of CEB by a factor of 0.86; that is, it decreases the CEB by 14% ($e^{-0.15}$), other things being equal. Fundamentalist Protestants and other Protestants do not seem to have significantly different levels of CEB as compared to Catholics. These results mean that the fertility differentials among Catholics and Protestants are shrinking. This echoes findings of previous research. But the fertility differentials among Catholics and other non-Christian religions do support my hypothesis on religion and fertility.

In models 2 and 3, I replace the current religious denomination variable with variables that represent people's religiosity. These variables are *frequency attending religious services* and *importance of religious beliefs in people's daily lives*, respectively. Apparently, people who reported that religious beliefs play an important role in their daily lives tend to have a higher level of CEB, whereas religious participation does not show a significant impact on fertility. A similar pattern also is found in models 4 and 5, after controlling the effect of religious denomination

Table 7.3 Poisson regression of CEB on religious affiliation, participation and beliefs: all male and female respondents: U.S., 2002

Variables	Model 1	Model 2	Model 3	Model 4	Model 5
Religious variables					
Current religious affiliation (ref. = Catholic)					
Fundamentalist Protestant	0.06			0.06	0.04
Other Protestant	0.04			0.05	0.03
Other non-Christian religion	−0.15*			−0.14*	−0.14*
Religiosity					
Frequency attending religious services		0.02		0.01	
Importance of religious beliefs			0.09***		0.08***
Demographic factors					
Age	0.05***	0.06***	0.05***	0.05***	0.06***
Gender (ref. = female)	−0.14***	−0.15***	−0.13***	−0.14***	−0.13***
Race and ethnicity (ref. = White)					
Hispanic	0.23***	0.21***	0.19***	0.23***	0.21***
Non-Hispanic black	0.25***	0.26***	0.23***	0.25***	0.22***
Non-Hispanic other	0.21*	0.16	0.15	0.21*	0.18
If R has ever been married	1.02***	1.02***	1.01***	1.01***	1.01***
Socioeconomic factors					
Highest degree R ever earned	−0.07***	−0.07***	−0.07***	−0.07***	−0.07***
Total combined family income	−0.02***	−0.03***	−0.02***	−0.03***	−0.02***
Constant	−1.55***	−1.54***	−1.70***	−1.58***	−1.72***
N	9,759	9,750	9,729	9,750	9,729
Prob > F	0.0000	0.0000	0.0000	0.0000	0.0000

Note: R refers to the respondent. *$p < 0.05$, **$p < 0.01$, ***$p < 0.001$ (two-tailed tests). Regression coefficients for nativity and ever work are not reported due to non-significant regression coefficients.

Sources: derived from NSFG Cycle 6 male and female datasets, 2002.

on fertility. The results can be interpreted as: over the total range of scale from 1 to 3 measuring religious beliefs, the expected CEB is multiplied by a factor of 1.1 ($e^{0.08}$), holding the other variables constant (see model 5). This finding means that the strength of religious beliefs does have a significantly positive impact on people's fertility, regardless to which religious denomination they belong. Unexpectedly, frequent churchgoers do not really show a significantly higher level of CEB. These findings corroborate hypothesis 2 but reject hypothesis 1.

Hypothesis 5 is tested by comparing the results of model 1 with models 4 and 5. Results show that fertility differentials among various groups do not change significantly, nor do the effects of other variables on fertility after taking religiosity into consideration. This finding does not support hypothesis 5, which ultimately undermines hypothesis 6. This finding means that fertility differentiation among various religious groups is not likely to be caused by different levels of religiosity among those religious groups. In other words, the effect of religious denomination on fertility is significant, net the influence of religiosity. Note that all results presented here are based on analyzing all male and female respondents.

In addition to the clear effects of religious denomination and religious beliefs on fertility, most of the covariates are influential as well. According to model 5, age has a significantly positive effect on fertility. From the age range of 15–45, the level of expected CEB increases by around 6% ($e^{0.06}$). Being a man decreases the level of expected CEB by 12% ($e^{-0.13}$), compared to being a woman, which emphasizes the significant gender effect on fertility. Having married increases the respondent's CEB by a factor of 2.8 ($e^{1.01}$), which indicates the imperative role of marriage in determining fertility. Race and ethnicity are found to influence fertility as well. Having a Hispanic background multiplies the number of children born to a respondent by a factor of 1.2 ($e^{0.21}$), holding the other independent variables constant. That is, Hispanics tend to have a CEB that is 20% higher as compared to whites, the reference group. Blacks and other racial groups also have a greater expected number of children than non-Hispanic whites. Education and income also have negative and significant effects on fertility. These results echo findings shown in Chapter 6 that focuses on the effects of demographic and socioeconomic characteristics on fertility.

Given the concern of underreporting births by younger men, in Table 7.4, I exclude male respondents who are 25 and younger. This part of the analysis falls in line with the analysis conducted in Chapter 6 that excludes younger males in the study. As compared to results shown in Table 7.3, in general, religious denomination, religious participation, and religious beliefs show similar effects on fertility after males 25 and younger are removed from the analysis. Such a consistency again supports hypothesis 2 and rejects hypotheses 1 and 5.

The major differences that occur when comparing the two groups with and without male respondents 25 and younger are the effects of two demographic covariates, namely, *gender* and *ever married*. They both show weaker effects when younger male respondents are dropped from the regression models. To illustrate, dropping younger male respondents from the analysis changes the negative effect of gender on fertility from 12% ($e^{0.13}$) to 8% ($e^{0.08}$). This means that being a man decreases the respondent's expected CEB by 12% when all respondents are examined. After

Table 7.4 Poisson regression of CEB on religious affiliation, participation and beliefs: male respondents 26 and over and all female respondents: U.S., 2002

Variables	Model 1	Model 2	Model 3	Model 4	Model 5
Religious variables					
Current religious affiliation (ref. = Catholic)					
Fundamentalist Protestant	0.05			0.05	0.03
Other Protestant	0.03			0.03	0.02
Other non-Christian religion	−0.16*			−0.15*	−0.16*
Religiosity		0.02		0.01	
Frequency attending religious services					
Importance of religious beliefs			0.09***		0.08***
Demographic factors					
Age	0.05***	0.05***	0.05***	0.05***	0.05***
Gender (ref. = female)	−0.10***	−0.10***	−0.09***	−0.10***	−0.08***
Race and ethnicity (ref. = White)					
Hispanic	0.20***	0.18***	0.17***	0.20***	0.18***
Non-Hispanic black	0.24***	0.24***	0.22***	0.23***	0.21***
Non-Hispanic other	0.18*	0.13	0.11	0.17	0.15
If R has ever been married	0.96***	0.96***	0.96***	0.96***	0.95***
Socioeconomic factors					
Highest degree R ever earned	−0.07***	−0.07***	−0.07***	−0.07***	−0.07***
Total combined family income	−0.02***	−0.02***	−0.02***	−0.03***	−0.02***
Constant	−1.31***	−1.32***	−1.48***	−1.35***	−1.48***
N	8,638	8,629	8,613	8,629	8,613
Prob > F	0.0000	0.0000	0.0000	0.0000	0.0000

Note: R refers to the respondent. *$p < 0.05$, **$p < 0.01$, ***$p < 0.001$ (two-tailed tests). Regression coefficients for *nativity* and *ever work* are not reported due to non-significant regression coefficients.

Sources: derived from NSFG Cycle 6 male and female datasets, 2002.

males 25 and younger are dropped from the analysis, being a man only decreases the respondent's CEB by 8%. After younger males are eliminated from the analysis, the effect of ever married on fertility alters from multiplying a factor of 2.8 ($e^{1.01}$) to 2.6 ($e^{0.95}$). These findings probably indicate that the gender and marriage effects on fertility tend to be weaker with an increasing age of male population. In general, the results suggest that the potential bias of underreporting births which may be caused by including younger males does not significantly changes the findings of this research.

Until now, I have tested hypotheses on the impacts of religious denominations and religiosity on fertility. Next, I will elaborate the models that contrast the effects of religion and religiosity on male and female fertility. I will show whether religion and religiosity impact men's and women's fertility differently. Models 1, 2 and 3 in Table 7.5 display Poisson regression results when analyzing all male and female respondents after incorporating the gender interaction terms. In model 1, I include variable *religious denomination*, the gender interaction terms, and demographic and socioeconomic variables to test hypothesis 6. I attempt to determine whether men's fertility differentials across religious groups are significantly different from those among women. As it can be seen, the gender interaction terms generated by religious denominations and the gender variable are not significant, which indicates that fertility differentials across religious groups do not vary substantially between men and women. This finding supports hypothesis 6. In models 2 and 3 of Table 7.5, I test whether the effects of religious participation and religious beliefs on fertility vary by gender after controlling for religious denominations and other factors, respectively. Neither of the gender interaction terms is observed as significant. These findings oppose hypotheses 2 and 4, which implies that stronger religiosity does not appear to increase women's fertility to a greater extent than men's, controlling for other factors.

Models 4 through 6 replicate the Poisson estimates of CEB in models 1, 2 and 3, excluding male respondents who are 25 and younger. There is no strong evidence showing that the effects of religious denominations and religiosity on fertility vary by gender. This result is consistent with findings based on analyzing all male and female respondents. These results suggest that underreporting of births that is associated with including fertility reports of younger men will not change extensively the estimated relationship between religious variables and fertility.

7.5 Conclusion and Discussion

In this chapter, I shed light on the effects of religious denomination and religiosity on male as compared to on female fertility. My findings echo the reports of Mosher and associates that fertility differentials across religious groups are shrinking in the United States (Mosher et al., 1986; National Center for Health Statistics, 2005; Westoff & Jone, 1979). My findings reflect this pattern by showing no significant fertility differences between fundamentalist Protestants, other Protestants, and

Table 7.5 Poisson regression of CEB on religious variables and gender interaction terms: U.S., 2002

Variables	All male and female respondents			Males 26 + and all females		
	Model 1	Model 2	Model 3	Model 4	Model 5	Model 6
Religious variables						
Current religious affiliation (ref. = Catholic)						
Fundamentalist Protestant	0.08	0.07	0.06	0.07	0.06	0.05
Other Protestant	0.02	0.01	0.01	0.01	0.00	−0.01
Other non-Christian religion	−0.12	−0.12	−0.11	−0.14	−0.13	−0.12
Religiosity						
Frequency attending religious services		0.02			0.02	
Importance of religious beliefs			0.09***			0.10***
Interaction terms						
Current religious affiliation (ref. = Catholic)						
Fundamentalist Protestant * gender	−0.04	−0.02	−0.04	−0.05	−0.03	−0.04
Other Protestant * gender	0.06	0.08	0.06	0.07	0.08	0.07
Other non-Christian religion * gender	−0.05	−0.04	−0.06	−0.05	−0.04	−0.06
Religiosity						
Frequency attending religious services * gender		−0.02			−0.02	
Importance of religious beliefs * gender			−0.01			−0.04

Table 7.5 (continued)

Variables	All male and female respondents			Males 26 + and all females		
	Model 1	Model 2	Model 3	Model 4	Model 5	Model 6
Demographic factors						
Age	0.06***	0.06***	0.06***	0.05***	0.05***	0.05***
Gender (ref. = female)	−0.15***	−0.12	−0.10	−0.10*	−0.06	0.00
Race and ethnicity (ref. = White)						
Hispanic	0.23***	0.23***	0.21***	0.20***	0.20***	0.18***
Non-Hispanic black	0.25***	0.25***	0.23***	0.24***	0.23***	0.21***
Non-Hispanic other	0.21*	0.21*	0.19	0.18	0.18	0.16
If R has ever been married	1.02***	1.02***	1.01***	0.96***	0.96***	0.95***
Socioeconomic factors						
Highest degree R ever earned	−0.07***	−0.07***	−0.07***	−0.07***	−0.07***	−0.07***
Total combined family income	−0.02***	−0.03***	−0.02***	−0.02***	−0.02***	−0.02***
Constant	−1.55***	−1.60***	−1.73***	−1.31***	−1.37***	−1.52***
N	9,759	9,750	9,729	8,638	8,629	8,629
Prob > F	0.0000	0.0000	0.0000	0.0000	0.0000	0.0000

Note: R refers to the respondent. *p < 0.05, **p < 0.01, ***p < 0.001 (two-tailed tests). Regression coefficients for *nativity* and *ever work* are not reported due to non-significant regression coefficients.
Sources: derived from NSFG Cycle 6 male and female datasets, 2002.

Catholics. Indeed, Catholics only show a significantly higher level of fertility when compared to other non-Christian religious people. I find that the shrinking pattern of fertility differentials across religious groups is shown among both religious men and women in the U.S. In other words, the effect of religious denomination on fertility does not vary by gender.

Compared to studies of religious denomination and fertility, religiosity has received far less attention in the literature. The findings demonstrated in this research, however, help to address this shortcoming. I find that even after controlling for religious denomination and demographic and socioeconomic factors, the importance of religious beliefs still exhibits a graded association with fertility among both men and women in the United States. This finding echoes the research results based on examining the European samples (Adsera, 2007; Ongaro, 2001; Westoff & Frejka, 2007) which shows that in Europe, religiosity plays a significant role in determining people's fertility. My research results along with findings of other research on the importance of religiosity in shaping fertility have a significant implication. That is, the substantially positive effect of religious beliefs on fertility must have something to do with the role of religion in guiding human behavior in terms of the issues of sexuality, cohabitation, marriage, and the function of family. This is because a number of religious doctrines are linked to delayed sexual debut and entry into cohabitation, and more positive attitudes toward entering marital unions and having children (Bearman & Bruckner, 2001; Lehrer, 2004; Marchena & Waite, 2001). As stated earlier in this chapter, Catholicism encourages large family size and is strongly against abortion. The Mormon theology emphasizes the central role of the family in the religious community. Both Protestants and Mormons have incentives to marry early and are oriented to home-based activities. As a result, people who consider religious beliefs important in daily lives are more likely to internalize their church teachings and thus to favor a large family size. This perhaps explains why religiosity is influential when determining both men's and women's fertility.

Interestingly, I do not find significant effects of religious participation on fertility among either men or women. In the preliminary analysis, I found that frequent churchgoers do display a higher level of fertility when demographic and socioeconomic factors are not controlled (findings are not shown but are available from the author upon request). After demographic and socioeconomic factors are controlled in the regression models, the significant effect of attending religious services disappears. So it is likely that fertility differences among people with different levels of religious participation are caused by variations in their demographic and socioeconomic compositions. Such a finding supports the characteristics hypothesis which states that demographic and socioeconomic characteristics rather than religion that differentiate people's fertility. The results suggest that religious beliefs might be a much better predictor of fertility than measures of the behavioral dimension of religiosity.

Compared to women's fertility, men's fertility is found to be impacted by religious denomination, participation, and beliefs in a similar manner. It is easy to understand why religious denominations determine men's and women's fertility in a similar way. But it is hard to interpret why religiosity does not show a stronger effect on female than on male fertility, which is a general pattern shown in previous studies. In reality, women also tend to be more religious than men. In the Cycle 6 dataset, 85% of female respondents reported themselves to be religious as compared to 79% of men. As already noted earlier, female respondents in the dataset also show a higher level of religiosity as compared to men when both measures of religiosity are taken into consideration. Thus, it is reasonable to assume that a higher level of religiosity should have a greater influence on women's than on men's fertility. Then how to explain the results of this research that religiosity impacts men's and women's fertility in a similar manner? Put differently, why are results of this research inconsistent to previous findings based on the European social context?

One possible explanation for this inconsistency is that previous studies seldom use significance tests to justify whether the effects of religious variables on male and female fertility are statistically different from each other. Male and female fertility differentials indicated by different regression coefficients shown in previous research could be caused by non-identical male and female sample sizes or standard errors in separate male and female regression models. The stronger effect of religiosity on female than on male fertility observed in previous literature probably is based on the larger regression coefficients estimated in the female models, which have not been statistically compared with those of males. To obtain more accurate results, applying statistical tests which take sample sizes and standard errors of the male and female datasets into consideration is necessary. Such statistical methods include generating gender interaction terms and Z statistical tests (Paternoster, Brame, Mazerolle, & Piquero, 1998). In this research, I statistically test the gender differences by incorporating the gender interaction terms, and I have not found significant gender differences in the relationship of religion, religiosity and fertility. I suspect that the inconsistent results shown in my research and previous studies may have been caused by whether applying statistical tests in the analyses. Another possible explanation of the inconsistency is that most of the literature cited in the current research is drawn from European societies. The American social context may lead to dissimilar findings regarding the effect of religiosity on fertility.

I recognize that the measurement of religious denominations and religiosity is very limited in the NSFG Cycle 6 dataset. Some important dimensions of religious participation and beliefs, such as dimensions of frequency of prayer or meditation, frequency of reading holy books, or beliefs in a God or an afterlife, are not available in the NSFG Cycle 6 dataset and are thus not considered in this research. Future research that includes these variables would improve current religious studies of male and female fertility. In addition, this article excludes those people without religious affiliations due to data constraint. The dataset does not present information of the respondent's religiosity if the respondent does not claim a religious denomination. It is possible that some people who are not affiliated with any religions are actively participating religious services. In order to fully address the impact of religiosity on fertility, future research needs to bring those people without religious affiliations into the analysis.

The influence of religion on men's and women's fertility also depends on the social contexts to which religious people belong. Future research could consider community- or country-level religious variables along with individual level variables to estimate religious influences on male and female fertility. Moreover, future research could consider examining the interaction effects between religious denominations and religiosity in determining fertility, which has been pointed out by some researchers (Lehrer, 2004; Marcum, 1988). The interaction effects between religious denominations and religiosity are shown to be non-significant in my preliminary analysis, which could be due to limited measures of religiosity in this study. Future research may consider including more sound measures of religiosity when such data become available.

In sum, religion is a very important institution spreading behavioral norms and providing social support for people. My analysis reveals that the fertility gap among religious groups is decreasing for both men and women, whereas religiosity, especially religious beliefs, demonstrates a significantly positive effect on fertility. Women do not exhibit a substantially greater likelihood of being influenced by either religious denominations or by religiosity than men. Thus, I conclude that religion and religiosity have significant impacts on both male and female fertility. However, religion and religiosity do not seem to be factors that differentiate male and female fertility among the U.S. religious population.

References

Adsera, A. (2007). Marital fertility and religion in Spain, 1985 and 1999. *Population Studies*, *60*(2), 205–221.

Ballard, B. N. (2004). *Patterns of intended and actual fertility among sub-groups of foreign-born and native-born Latinas*. College Station, TX: Texas A&M University.

Barro, R. J., & McCleary, R. M. (2003). Religion and economic growth across countries. *American Sociological Review*, *68*, 760–781.

Bearman, P. S., & Bruckner, H. (2001). Promising the future: virginity pledges and first intercourse. *American Journal of Sociology*, *106*(4), 859–912.

Berrington, A. (2001). Transition to adulthood in Britain. In M. Corijn & E. Klijzing (Eds.), *Transition in adulthood in Europe* (pp. 67–102). Dordrecht: Kluwer Academic Publisher.

Bongaarts, J. (1982). The fertility-inhibiting effects of the intermediate fertility variables. *Studies in Family Planning*, *13*(6), 179–189.

Bongaarts, J., & Watkins, S. S. (1996). Social interaction and contemporary fertility transition. *Population and Development Review*, *22*(4), 639–682.

Bouvier, L. F., & Rao, S. L. N. (1975). *Socioreligious factors in fertility decline*. Cambridge, MA: Ballinger.

Chamie, J. (1981). *Religion and fertility: Arab Christian-Muslim differentials*. Cambridge: Cambridge University Press.

Coale, A. J., & Trussell, J. (1974). Model fertility schedules: Variations in the age structure of childbearing in human populations. *Population Studies*, *44*(2), 203–213.

Coale, A. J., & Watkins, S. S. (1986). *The decline of fertility in Europe*. Princeton, NJ: Princeton University Press.

Corijn, M. (2001). Transition to adulthood in Flanders (Belgium). In M. Corijn & E. Klijzing (Eds.), *Transition in adulthood in Europe* (pp. 103–130). Dordrecht: Kluwer Academic Publisher.

Corijn, M., & Klijzing, E. (2001). *Transitions to adulthood in Europe*. New York, NY: Kluwer Academic Publishers.

De Jong, G. F. (1965). Religious fundamentalism, socioeconomic status and fertility attitudes in the Southern Appalachians. *Demography*, *2*, 540–548.

Ellison, C., Echevarria, S., & Smith, B. (2005). Religion and abortion attitudes among U.S. Hispanics: Findings from the 1990 Latino national political survey. *Social Science Quarterly*, *86*(1), 192–208.

Freedman, R., Whelpton, P. K., & Smith, J. W. (1961). Socio-economic factors in religious differentials in Fertility. *American Sociological Review*, *26*(4), 608–614.

Goldscheider, C. (1971). *Population, modernization and social structure*. Boston, MA: Little, Brown and Co.

Goldscheider, F. K., & Goldscheider, C. (1993). *Leaving home before marriage: Ethnicity, familism and generational relationships*. Madison, WI: University of Wisconsin Press.

Goldscheider, C., & Uhlenberg, P. R. (1969). Minority group status and fertility. *American Journal of Sociology*, *74*(4), 361–372.

Hervitz, H. M. (1985). Selectivity, adaptation, or disruption? A comparison of alternative hypotheses on the effects of migration on fertility: The case of Brazil. *International Migration Review*, *19*(2), 293–317.

Jaffe, A. J., & Cullen, R. M. (1975). Fertility of the Puerto Rican origin population-Mainland United States and Puerto Rico: 1970. *International Migration Review*, *9*(2), 193–209.

Janssen, S. G., & Hauser, R. M. (1981). Religion, socialization, and fertility. *Demography*, *18*(4), 511–528.

Johnson-Hanks, J. (2006). On the politics and practice of Muslim fertility – Comparative evidence from West Africa. *Medical Anthropology Quarterly*, *20*(1), 12–30.

Jurecki-Tiller, M. (2004). *The Influence of Religion on Childbearing: Fertility, Reproductive Biology and Belief in the Church of Jesus Christ of Latter-Day Saints*. Unpublished Dissertation, The State University of New York at Buffalo, Buffalo.

Knodel, J., Gray, R. S., Sriwatchrin, P., & Peracca, S. (1999). Religion and reproduction: Muslims in Buddhist Thailand. *Population Studies*, *53*(2), 149–164.

Lehrer, E. L. (1996). The role of the husband's religious affiliation in the economic and demographic behavior of families. *Journal for the Scientific Study of Religion*, *35*(2), 145–155.

Lehrer, E. L. (2004). Religion as a determinant of economic and demographic behavior in the United States. *Population and Development Review*, *30*(4), 707–726.

Marchena, E., & Waite, L. J. (2001). Marriage and Childbearing Attitudes in Late Adolescence: Gender, Race and Ethnic Differences. Annual Meeting of the Population Association of America

Marcum, J. P. (1981). Explaining fertility differentials among U.S. *Protestants, Social Forces*, *60*(2), 532–543.

Marcum, J. P. (1988). Religious affiliation, participation and fertility: A cautionary note. *Journal for the Scientific Study of Religion*, *27*(4), 621–629.

McQuillan, K. (2004). When does religion influence fertility? *Population and Development Review*, *30*(1), 25–56.

Montgomery, M. R., & Casterline, J. B. (1996). Social learning, social influence, and new models of fertility. *Population and Development Review*, *22*, 151–175.

Mosher, W. D., & Hendershot, G. E. (1984). Religious affiliation and the fertility of married couples. *Journal of Marriage and Family*, *46*(3), 671–677.

Mosher, W. D., Johnson, D. P., & Horn, M. C. (1986). Religion and fertility in the United States: The importance of marriage patterns and Hispanic origin. *Demography*, *23*(3), 367–379.

Mosher, W. D., Williams, L. B., & Johnson, D. P. (1992). Religion and fertility in the United States: New patterns. *Demography*, *29*(3), 199–214.

Myers, S. M. (1996). An interactive model of religiosity inheritance: The importance of family context. *American Sociological Review*, *61*, 858–866.

National Center for Health Statistics. (2005). *Fertility, Family Planning and Reproductive Health of US Women: Data from the 2002 National Survey of Family Growth*. Hyattsville, Maryland, MD.

Ongaro, F. (2001). Transition to adulthood in Italy. In M. Corijn & E. Klijzing (Eds.), *Transition in adulthood in Europe* (pp. 173–207). Dordrecht: Kluwer Academic Publisher.
Paternoster, B., Brame, R., Mazerolle, P., & Piquero, A. (1998). Using the correct statistical test for the equality of regression coefficients. *Criminology*, *36*(4), 859–866.
Poston, D. L. J. (1990). Voluntary and involuntary childlessness among Catholic and Non-Catholic women: Are the patterns converging? *Social Biology*, *37*(3&4), 251–265.
Poston, D. L. J., Chang, C. -F., & Dan, H. (2006). Fertility differences between the majority and minority nationality groups in China *Population Research and Policy Review*, *26*, 67–101.
Preiffer, C., & Nowak, V. (2001). Transition to adulthood in Austria. In M. Corijn & E. Klijzing (Eds.), *Transition in adulthood in Europe* (pp. 43–66). Dordrecht: Kluwer Academic Publisher.
Ryder, N. (1974). Comment. In T. W. Schultz (Ed.), *Economics of the family* (pp. 76–80). Chicago: University of Chicago Press.
Saenz, R., & Morales, M. C. (2005). Demography of race and ethnicity. In J. Poston, L. Dudley, & M. Micklin (Eds.), *Handbook of population*. New York, NY: Academics/Kluwers.
Sander, W. (1992). Catholicism and the economics of fertility. *Population Studies*, *46*(3), 477–489.
Sander, W. (1993). Catholicism and marriage in the United States. *Demography*, *30*(3), 373–384.
Singley, S. G., & Landale, N. S. (1998). Incorporating origin and process in migration fertility frameworks: The case of Puerto Rican women. *Social Forces*, *76*(4), 1437–1464.
Watkins, S. C. (1992). *From provinces into nations: Demographic integration in Western Europe, 1870–1960*. Princeton, NJ: Princeton University Press.
Westoff, C. F., & Frejka, T. (2007). Fertility and religiousness among European Muslims. *Population and Development Review*, *33*, 785–809.
Westoff, C. F., & Jone, E. F. (1979). The end of "Catholic" fertility. *Demography*, *16*(2), 209–217.
Xie, Y., & Pimentel, E. E. (1992). Age patterns of marital fertility: Revising the Coale-Trussell method. *Journal of the American Statistical Association*, *87*(420), 977–984.
Yeatman, S. E., & Trinitapoli, J. (2007). *Beyond Denomination: New Tests of Whether and How Religion Matters for Family Planning*. Paper presented at the Annual Meetings of Population Association of America New York City.

Chapter 8
The Influence of Cohabitation on Male and Female Fertility

With an increasing number of cohabiters in the United States and other industrialized countries, the role of cohabitation in fertility and family formation has attracted a considerable attention of family scholars in a variety of fields. When it comes to fertility, in particular, previous studies have documented a prominent role of cohabitation in determining women's childbearing results. Previous studies, however, have seldom examined the influence of cohabitation on men's fertility results. In this chapter, I attempt to bring male fertility into the analysis of cohabitation and fertility. Given the racial and ethnic differences shown in prior research and the entangled relationships between cohabitation, one's socioeconomic factors, family-background characteristics and the proximate determinants in determining fertility, the analysis of this chapter also takes race and ethnicity and the interaction effects between cohabitation and other covariates into consideration. The chapter examines two subject matters: (1) how cohabitation influences male and female fertility through mediating with one's socioeconomic characteristics, the family-background characteristics and the proximate determinants; (2) how the effect of cohabitation on male and female fertility varies across racial and ethnic groups when the interaction effects between cohabitation and other covariates are taken into consideration.

Before I conduct the empirical analysis, I will first review prior literature on cohabitation and fertility in the next a few subsections of the chapter. These previous studies offer a theoretical guidance to this current research. Based on findings of the reviewed work, I then proposed several research hypotheses on cohabitation and male and female fertility for testing.

8.1 Linking Cohabitation and Female Childbearing

Previous literature has documented a strong association between premarital cohabitation and female childbearing. Empirical evidence comes from the comparison results of cohabiters' fertility with those of singles and married couples. Bachrach (1987) finds that cohabiting women have a higher expected rate of fertility than non-cohabiting singles. In regard to the comparison analyses of fertility among married couples and cohabiters, researchers reveal that female cohabiters' fertility was once

L. Zhang, *Male Fertility Patterns and Determinants*, The Springer Series on Demographic Methods and Population Analysis 27, DOI 10.1007/978-90-481-8939-7_8,

lower than that of married couples; it then began to catch up to fertility of married women. For instance, in the United States, Rindfuss and VandenHeuvel (1990) find that in the late 1970s, by age 25, female cohabiters' fertility was more similar to singles than married couples. This pattern continued to the 1980s, shown in Bachrach's study (1987) of a lower fertility level among cohabiting couples than married couples. Nevertheless, by the early 1990s, the number of births to cohabiting women is found to be nearer that of married women. This trend is also documented in Raley's (2001) study when examining the 1995 National Survey and Family Growth (NSFG) dataset and the 1987–1988 National Survey of Families and Households (NSFH). Similar fertility levels for cohabiting women and married women are also shown in the literature when examining marital fertility in Europe in the 1980s (Blanc, 1984; Carlson, 1986). The increasing similarity in fertility among cohabiting and married women is believed to be due to the rising proportions of women who bear children in cohabiting households (Bumpass & Sweet, 1989; Cherlin, 1992). Based on findings of previous studies, I propose that a positive effect of cohabitation on fertility also exists among males. So I set for the following two hypotheses for testing:

Hypothesis 1: Cohabitation has a positive effect on fertility, controlling for other factors. And,

Hypothesis 2: The positive effect of cohabitation on fertility does not vary by gender.

8.2 Racial and Ethnic Differences in the Relationship of Cohabitation and Fertility

In the social context of the United States, racial and ethnic differences are also found in the relationship of cohabitation and fertility. In terms of union formation for childbearing, researchers find that the racial and ethnic differences do exist among sub-populations. To illustrate, there are greater proportions of Hispanics and blacks than whites who choose cohabitation as their first unions (Clarkberg, 1999; Loomis & Landale, 1994). Moreover, whites are more likely to be in a trial marriage type of cohabitation, whereas blacks tend to be in a substitute for marriage type of cohabitation (Casper & Sayer, 2000). In addition, blacks and Hispanics are more likely to stay in nonmarital unions for a longer period of time as compared to whites due to their greater level of economic disadvantage (Brown, 2000; Goldstein & Kenney, 2001; Manning, 1995).

When it comes to childbearing, black and Hispanic women show more tolerance towards having children outside of marriage. Hispanic and black women are also more likely to conceive a child in cohabitation households than whites (Bachu, 1999; Fields & Casper, 2001; Manning, 2001; Wildsmith & Raley, 2006). The proportion of children born to cohabiting Hispanic and black parents largely surpasses that among cohabiting white couples (Smock & Manning, 2004). Moreover, Hispanic women are found to be more inclined than white and black women to have intended pregnancies in cohabitation unions (Manning, 2001; Musick, 2002). Prior research also shows that when women become pregnant while cohabiting, blacks and Hispanics are three and two times more likely, respectively, than whites to stay in cohabiting unions with their partners even after a birth occurs (Manning, 2001). According to these results, I propose the following hypothesis:

Hypothesis 3: Blacks and Hispanics are more similar than different as compared to whites in the cohabitation and fertility relationship, controlling for other factors.

8.3 Socioeconomic Status, Family-Background Characteristics, and Nonmarital Fertility

Of relevance to the racial and ethnic differences in cohabitation and childbearing is the evidence from prior literature that suggests an entangled relationship between socioeconomic status, family-background characteristics and cohabitation (Wildsmith & Raley, 2006). As far as socioeconomic status is concerned, prior analyses show that there are strong links between education, income, labor force participation and women's cohabitation and childbearing outcome. For instance, women with less education are found to be more likely to cohabit than those with higher education (Seltzer, 2004). Poor women are less likely to marry and more likely to cohabit and to have nonmarital births than women in relatively more advantaged socioeconomic status (C. Bachrach, Hindin, & Thomson, 2000; Wildsmith & Raley, 2006). Women's longer periods of employment are also found negatively associated with having premarital births (Budig, 2003).

Besides socioeconomic factors, links between family-background characteristics, cohabitation and childbearing are also revealed by previous analyses. Family-background characteristics are characterized by the family structure and parental economic resources. The family structure is often classified as the single-parent family or the intact family structure. Parental economic resources are often measured by parental educational attainments which represent human and social capital that is invested in children. Researchers find that children with greater investment from their parents are able to obtain greater social achievements than those with less parental investment (Bianchi & Robinson, 1997). The lack of parental economic resources often increases the risk of cohabiting and having births in nonmarital unions (Manning, 1995). The family structure matters in the cohabitation and fertility relationship because of the following reasons: first, single parents exert less supervision and control than married parents on their children (Thomson, McLanahan, & Curtin, 1992). Consequently, individuals from single-parent families are more likely to cohabit and to give birth in nonmarital unions (Althaus, 1997; Berrington & Diamond, 1999; McLanahan & Sandefur, 1994; Wildsmith & Raley, 2006). Second, attitudes and behaviors transferred from parents is an important mechanism that regulates an individual's subsequent fertility and family formation patterns. Following this rationale, researchers argue that children in single-parent families are more likely to choose cohabitation rather than marriage. This is because children in single-parent families are likely to inherit characteristics from their parents. These characteristics are often linked to nontraditional attitudes towards marriage and childbearing (Kamp Dush, Cohan, & Amato, 2003), which increases the likelihood of cohabiting and giving birth outside of marriage. Socioeconomic status and family characteristics are also believed to be able to partially explain the fertility differentials among cohabiters across racial and ethnic groups (Manning, 1995; Musick, 2002). Given the results presented in the above findings, I propose that the socioeconomic factors and family-background characteristics influence the effect of cohabitation on fertility. Put differently, the effect of cohabitation on fertility mediates with one's socioeconomic status and family-background characteristics. My hypotheses regarding cohabitation and socioeconomic status are proposed as follows:

Hypothesis 4: The positive effect of cohabitation on fertility depends on one's educational attainment; the higher the level of one's education, the weaker the effect of cohabitation on fertility.

Hypothesis 5: The positive effect of cohabitation on fertility mediates with one's income; the higher the income, the weaker the effect of cohabitation on fertility.

Hypothesis 6: The positive effect of cohabitation on fertility varies by one's employment status. The positive effect of cohabitation on fertility is stronger among unemployed than employed individuals, controlling for other factors.

The following two hypotheses regard the interaction effects between cohabitation and family-background characteristics on fertility.

Hypothesis 7: One's cohabitation experience mediates with his/her parental educational attainment. The effect of cohabitation on fertility diminishes with an increasing level of parental education. And,

Hypothesis 8: The effect of cohabitation on fertility varies by one's family structure. The cohabitation effect on fertility should be weaker among those who lived in intact families before age 18 than that among those who did not.

8.4 The Proximate Determinants, Cohabitation and Fertility

Previous studies also suggest that the proximate determinants can mediate with cohabitation to determine childbearing. According to Caldwell (1982), the primary proximate determinants include delayed marriage, the use of contraception, induced abortion and postpartum infecundability. Along with the secondary proximate determinants, such as waiting time to conception, risk of intrauterine mortality and onset of permanent sterility, the proximate determinants account for over 90% of fertility variation at the societal level (Knodel, Chamratrithirong, & Debavalya, 1987). The interaction effect of cohabitation and the proximate determinants have indeed been documented in previous analyses. Using the interaction effect between cohabitation and marriage as an example, Bachrach (1987) shows that cohabiting women with a marriage experience are less likely to use contraceptives and more inclined to have planned births in cohabitation unions than those with no marriage experience. Such an interaction effect is found to vary across racial and ethnic groups because timing of marriage varies considerably among different racial and ethnic groups. Cherlin (1992) finds that black women tend to start and stop their childbearing earlier and get married later than white women. As a consequence, a higher percentage of births occur to young and unmarried black parents as compared to their white counterparts. Due to findings of previous research, in this chapter, I consider the proximate determinants and examine how they interact with cohabitation to determine fertility. In this analysis, the proximate determinants are measured by number of marriages, age at first sexual intercourse and whether one had conducted a sterilization operation. These measures are considered as the proxies of the proximate determinants. The hypotheses regarding cohabitation, the proximate determinants and fertility are proposed as follows:

Hypothesis 9: Cohabitation mediates with the number of marriages to affect one's fertility outcome. Specifically, a greater number of marriages decreases the effect of cohabitation on fertility.

Hypothesis 10: The influence of cohabitation on fertility decreases with an increasing age at first sex, controlling for other factors. And,

Hypothesis 11: The effect of cohabitation on fertility depends on whether one had a sterilization operation. Cohabitation has a stronger positive effect on those who never had a sterilization operation than those who became sterilized, controlling for other factors.

In the next section of the chapter, I present data, variables and methods used to test the proposed hypotheses.

8.5 Data, Variables and Methods

For this study, data are from the 2002 wave of the National Survey of Family Growth (NSFG). In my analysis, I combine female and male datasets together for the purpose of generating gender interaction terms, which allows me to test whether male and female fertility outcomes are affected by cohabitation in significantly different ways. As indicated earlier, considering underreporting of births by younger men in the NSFG dataset revealed by Rendall and associates (Rendall et al., 2006), I break the analysis into two parts. The first part contains all male and female respondents and the second part excludes males who are 25 years of age and younger. Results based on examining the two sets of data are compared and contrasted. I assume that the results based on examining the dataset which excludes younger men should have a higher validity since it reduces the potential bias that may be caused by underreporting of births by younger men.

The dependent variable in this research representing fertility outcome is measured by the number of children ever born (CEB) to a male or a female respondent. The primary independent variable, cohabitation, is measured by two variables. The first variable is *ever cohabited,* which is a dummy variable based on the NSFG question regarding whether the respondent has ever lived with a nonmarital partner. It is coded as "1" if the respondent has ever cohabited and "0" if otherwise. It is worth mentioning that in the NSFG questionnaire, only cohabitation experience with partners of the opposite sex is considered. In other words, the cohabitation questions in the 2002 NSFG questionnaire do not allow researchers to examine cohabitation patterns of homosexuals.

The second cohabitation variable, *cohabitation experience*, comes from the NSFG questions asking whether the respondent had ever cohabited and whether the respondent had cohabited only with his/her spouse or has cohabited with partners he/she never married. I generate a variable *cohabitation experience* by combining information based on the respondent's answers to both questions. I code the variable *cohabitation experience* as "1" if the respondent has never cohabited, "2" if the respondent cohabited only with his/her spouse(s) before marriage and "3" if the respondent cohabited with other partners that the respondent has never married. Respondents with no cohabitation experience are classified as the reference category.

In addition to the above variables, I also include variables representing the respondent's demographic characteristics, socioeconomic status, family-background characteristics, and several proximate determinant variables. The demographic factors controlled in this research are age, gender, nativity, and metropolitan residence, which have been revealed as important factors influencing fertility (Ballard, 2004; Bloom & Trussell, 1984; Chang, Freedman, & Sun, 1987; Ellison, Echevarria, & Smith, 2005; Lehrer, 1996; R.R. Rindfuss, Morgan, & Swicegood, 1988; Sander, 1992). The variables measuring the respondent's socioeconomic status are *education, total combined family income*, and *labor force participation.* The labor force participation variable is operationalized by asking whether the respondent had worked full time for more than 6 months. Family-background characteristics are measured by variables *mother's education, father's education, whether the respondent has lived in an intact family till age* 18, and *whether the respondent was raised with a certain religious affiliation at age* 14. The religious variable is included in this analysis because religion is considered as an important means of socialization. Religion is also found to positively influence fertility through family formation and timing of giving first birth (Bloom & Trussell, 1984; Jurecki-Tiller, 2004; McLanahan & Bumpass, 1988; Mosher, Johnson, & Horn, 1986; R.R. Rindfuss et al., 1988).

The proximate determinant variables used in this research are *number of times the respondent has been married*, *age at first sexual intercourse* and *whether the respondent had a sterilization operation.* Ideally, variables representing age at first marriage, contraceptive use and postpartum infecundability should be used as measures of the proximate determinants. In the NSFG dataset, however, these variables are not readily available for male respondents. I thus decided to use variables that are as close as to the ideal measures of the proximate determinants. Age at first sexual intercourse is used because it indicates the sexual maturity of an individual, which influences an individual's completed fertility in later ages. Prior research shows women who begin sexual activities at younger ages tend to have a high premarital childbearing rate and are more likely to marry young (Miller & Heaton, 1991). Sterilization is included as a proximate determinant because having a sterilization operation has a similar effect on fertility behavior as contraceptive use. The number of times the respondent has been married is used as a measure of the marriage effect on childbearing.

Besides the above variables, I have also generated a gender interaction term by multiplying the gender variable with the cohabitation variable. The purpose of generating the gender interaction variable is to examine whether males and females have significantly different fertility results due to cohabitation. Descriptive information for all variables discussed is presented in Tables 8.1 and 8.2.

Because CEB is a count variable, Poisson regression is the statistical procedure used to conduct the analysis. The Poisson regression model is written as:

$$\mu_i = \exp\left(a + X_{1i}b_1 + X_{2i}b_2 + \ldots + X_{ki}b_k\right) \quad (1)$$

Where μ_i is the mean of the distribution, which is estimated from observed characteristics of the independent variables; a is the constant; b_i represents deviation from the mean of the omitted category, which is the reference group. The X variables are related to μ nonlinearly. In this case, μ_i is the expected number of children born to a respondent based on the cohabitation variable, socioeconomic status and so forth. All cases in regression models are weighted based on the final weights of each sample given by the NSFG.

8.6 Results

8.6.1 Descriptive Results

Tables 8.1 and 8.2 present descriptive information of variables included in the analysis. Table 8.1 shows the descriptive information of variables by gender and Table 8.2 focuses on demonstrating the descriptive results by racial and ethnic groups. As the tables show, the average CEB is 1.3 for women with a standard deviation of 0.03. The average CEB for men is 1.1 with a standard deviation of 0.04. On average, female respondents reported a greater number of children than their male counterparts. However, there is a greater variation in male than in female fertility. When the racial and ethnic differences in fertility are considered, for all male and female respondents, Hispanics show the highest average level of CEB (1.5), followed by blacks (1.4) and whites have reported the lowest fertility (1.1) (see Table 8.2).

In terms of the respondent's cohabitation experience, there is a slightly higher percentage of female than male respondents who reported having had a cohabitation experience (50 versus 48.8%). When it comes to the racial and ethnic differences,

Table 8.1 Descriptive statistics for dependent, independent and control variables by gender: U.S., 2002

Variables	Male (all respondents)			Male (26 and over)			Female (all respondents)		
	Mean (or %)	S.E.	N	Mean (or %)	S.E.	N	Mean (or %)	S.E.	N
Dependent variable									
CEB	1.1	0.04	4,117	1.5	0.04	2,622	1.3[a]	0.03	7,642
Independent variables									
Cohabitation variables									
If ever cohabited			4,927			2,744			7,643
Yes	48.8			63.5			50.0		
No	51.2			36.5			50.0		
Cohabitation experience			4,927			2,744			7,636
Never cohabited	51.2			36.5			49.9		
Only cohabited with spouse(s)	19.2			28.0			30.3		
Cohabited with partners R never Married	29.6			35.4			19.8		
Control variables									
Demographic factors									
Age (mean)	29.8	0.23	4,927	35.3	0.16	2,744	30.0	0.17	7,643
Race and ethnicity			4,927			2,744			7,643
Hispanic	16.7			16.2			14.8		
Non-Hispanic white	65.4			67.0			64.7		
Non-Hispanic black	11.9			10.9			14.0		
Non-Hispanic other	6.0			5.9			5.6		
Nativity-if foreign born			4,925			2,733			7,643
Native born	84.7			83.3			85.7		
Foreign born	15.3			16.7			14.3		
Metropolitan residence			4,927						
Yes	81.4			80.8		2,744	82.3		7,643
No	18.6			19.2			17.7		

Table 8.1 (continued)

Variables	Male (all respondents)			Male (26 and over)			Female (all respondents)		
	Mean (or %)	S.E.	N	Mean (or %)	S.E.	N	Mean (or %)	S.E.	N
Socioeconomic factors									
R's highest education			4,927			2,744			7,643
Less than high school	22.9			15.6			21.2		
High school graduate	31.5			33.5			28.3		
Some college/college	26.1			25.7			30.4		
University and above	19.5			25.3			20.1		
If R ever worked full time for 6+ months			4,925			2,742			7,636
Yes	79.1			96.7			74.1		
No	20.9			3.3			25.9		
Combined family income			4,927			2,744			7,643
$24,999 and under	27.4			23.1			33.1		
$25,000–$49,999	33.3			35.4			30.3		
$50,000–$74,999	18.5			19.7			18.9		
$75,000 and above	20.8			21.8			17.7		
Socialization factors									
Mother's education			4,902			2,729			7,593
Less than high school	21.4			24.2			24.1		
High school graduate	38.0			40.9			36.1		
Some college/college	20.9			17.9			21.7		
University and above	20.1			17.0			18.1		
Father's education			4,505			2,504			6,896
Less than high school	23.9			27.7			23.7		
High school graduate	30.7			31.1			31.5		
Some college/college	19.1			16.6			19.0		
University and above	26.3			24.7			25.8		

Table 8.1 (continued)

Variables	Male (all respondents)			Male (26 and over)			Female (all respondents)		
	Mean (or %)	S.E.	N	Mean (or %)	S.E.	N	Mean (or %)	S.E.	N
Lived in intact family till 18			4,927			2,744			7,643
Yes	68.4			70.8			65.3		
No	31.6			29.2			34.7		
If raised up with a religious affiliation	81.3		4,910	83.7		2,734	85.9		7,620
Yes									
No	18.7			17.3			14.1		
Proximate determinants									
Number of times R has been married	0.62	0.02	4,927	0.90	0.02	2,744	0.72	0.02	7,643
If R ever had sterilization operation			4,925			2,742			7,643
Yes	6.4			9.8			18.2		
No	93.6			90.2			81.8		
Age at 1st sexual intercourse	17.0	0.08	4,108	17.4	0.1	2,612	17.3	0.06	6,785

Note: some sub-categories may not add up to 100% due to rounding. All cases are weighted in this table.
[a]The CEB value for women who are 26 and over is 1.8 with a standard deviation of 0.04.
Sources: derived from NSFG Cycle 6 male and female datasets, 2002.

Table 8.2 Descriptive statistics for dependent, independent and control variables by race and ethnicity: U.S., 2002

Variables	Whites Mean (or %)	Whites S.E.	Whites N	Hispanics Mean (or %)	Hispanics S.E.	Hispanics N	Blacks Mean (or %)	Blacks S.E.	Blacks N
Dependent variable									
CEB	1.1	0.04	6,231	1.5	0.05	2,547	1.4	0.05	2,362
Independent variables									
Cohabitation variables									
If ever cohabited			6,740			2,712			2,460
Yes	49.9			48.0			51.6		
No	50.1			51.2			48.4		
Cohabitation experience			6,739			2,709			2,458
Never cohabited	50.1			51.9			48.3		
Only cohabited with spouse(s)	26.2			24.6			19.7		
Cohabited with partners R never married	23.7			23.4			31.9		
Control variables									
Demographic factors									
Age (mean)	30.3	0.19	6,740	28.9	0.25	2,712	29.3	0.30	2,460
Nativity-if foreign born			6,728			2,699			2,452
Native born	95.9			51.8			89.6		
Foreign born	4.1			48.2			10.4		
Metropolitan residence			6,740						
Yes	78.0			92.6		2,712	90.4		2,460
No	22.0			7.4			9.6		
Socioeconomic factors									
R's highest education			6,740			2,712			2,460
Less than high school	17.1			41.6			24.9		
High school graduate	29.1			30.7			35.6		
Some college/college	29.2			19.2			27.5		
University and above	24.6			3.5			12.0		

Table 8.2 (continued)

Variables	Whites			Hispanics			Blacks		
	Mean (or %)	S.E.	N	Mean (or %)	S.E.	N	Mean (or %)	S.E.	N
If R ever worked full time for 6+ months			6,736			2,709			2,459
Yes	78.1			74.1			75.3		
No	21.9			25.9			24.7		
Combined family income			6,740			2,712			2,460
$24,999 and under	22.7			46.5			45.9		
$25,000–$49,999	31.8			33.4			29.9		
$50,000–$74,999	21.5			12.2			13.7		
$75,000 and above	24.0			7.9			10.5		
Socialization factors									
Mother's education			6,694			2,699			2,450
Less than high school	13.0			59.1			23.8		
High school graduate	41.1			22.1			38.5		
Some college/college	23.7			11.9			22.8		
University and above	22.2			6.9			14.9		
Father's education			6,350			2,408			2,036
Less than high school	15.6			58.5			27.1		
High school graduate	32.9			20.8			37.9		
Some college/college	20.8			10.9			19.1		
University and above	30.7			9.7			16.0		
Lived in intact family till 18			6,469			2,607			2,323
Yes	71.7			70.6			53.4		
No	28.3			29.4			46.6		
If raised up with a religious affiliation			6,722			2,704			2,447
Yes	90.7			96.2			94.8		
No	9.3			3.8			5.2		

Table 8.2 (continued)

Variables	Whites			Hispanics			Blacks		
	Mean (or %)	S.E.	N	Mean (or %)	S.E.	N	Mean (or %)	S.E.	N
Proximate determinants									
Number of times R has been married	0.73	0.02	6,740	0.61	0.02	2,712	0.72	0.02	7,643
If R ever had sterilization operation			6,739			2,712			2,459
Yes	12.7			11.2			13.9		
No	87.3			88.8			86.1		
Age at 1st sexual intercourse	17.2	0.06	5,754	17.3	0.10	2,392	15.9	0.10	2,210

Note: some sub-categories may not add up to 100% due to rounding. All cases are weighted in this table.
[a]The CEB value for women who are 26 and over is 1.8 with a standard deviation of 0.04.
Sources: derived from NSFG Cycle 6 male and female datasets, 2002.

according to Table 8.2, there is a higher percentage of blacks who reported having had a cohabitation experience as compared to non-Hispanic whites and Hispanics (51.6, 49.9 and 48%, respectively). If the respondent's cohabitation experience is further classified as having only cohabited with spouses before marriage and having cohabited with partners the respondent had never married, gender and racial and ethnic differences again emerge. The results show that approximately 30.0% of the female respondents reported a cohabitation experience only with their husbands, which account for 60% of all women who reported a cohabitation experience. These are respondents who have converted their cohabitation partnerships to marriages. The rest of the 19.8% of female respondents claimed that they had cohabited with other partner(s) whom they had never married. This group of women accounts for 40% of all female respondents with a cohabitation experience. As far as the male respondents are concerned, there is a higher percentage (29.6%) of men who did not transform their cohabitation partnerships to marriages as compared to those men who had converted their cohabitation partnerships to marriages (19.2%). These findings suggest that women are probably more likely to report their cohabitation relationships having been transformed to marriages than their male counterparts. Again, it needs to be pointed out here that the male and female respondents in the dataset are not husbands and wives. They are randomly selected individuals from different households.

If race and ethnicity is taken into consideration, it is observed that there is a higher percentage of blacks who reported having had cohabited with partners they had never married as compared to non-Hispanic whites and Hispanics (see Table 8.2). Thus, blacks perhaps have a lower chance to convert their cohabitation relationships to marriages as compared to other racial and ethnic groups.

As far as the demographic characteristics of the respondents, the majority of the respondents in the dataset are composed by non-Hispanic whites (approximately 65%). The rest around 16, 12 and 6% of the samples are Hispanics, non-Hispanic blacks and other non-Hispanic racial and ethnic groups, respectively. If gender is further taken into consideration, there is a slightly higher percentage of male than female respondents who claimed themselves as Hispanics (17 versus 15%). There is also a slightly higher percentage of black females than males (14.0 versus 11.9%) in the dataset. The major racial and ethnic difference shown in the respondent's demographic characteristics is their nativity. Only 4.1% of non-Hispanic whites reported themselves as foreign born, whereas 10.4% of blacks and 48.2% of Hispanics reported themselves as foreign born. The finding suggests that the Hispanic samples in the NSFG Cycle 6 dataset are highly represented by foreign-born individuals. Another racial and ethnic difference is shown in terms of the respondent's residence. As it is shown in Table 8.2, non-Hispanic whites are more likely to reside in non-MSAs as compared to Hispanics and blacks.

As regard to the respondent's socioeconomic status, the results indicate that Hispanics and blacks are in a more socioeconomically disadvantaged position than non-Hispanic whites. In particular, there are over 40% of Hispanics without high school diplomas. Almost half of the Hispanic and black respondents reported having a combined family income in 2001 lower than $25,000. Such racial and ethnic differentials in socioeconomic status may have an impact on the respondent's cohabitation and childbearing patterns.

The socioeconomic differentials by gender and race and ethnicity are also shown in the respondent's educational attainment. Data show that a slightly higher percentage of female respondents reported having advanced educational degrees than their male counterparts. Interestingly, when the respondent's educational attainments are compared to those of their parents, there does not seem to be a significant improvement in educational attainments of these two generations. When race and ethnicity are taken into consideration, Hispanics reported considerably lower levels of educational attainments than blacks and non-Hispanic whites. This pattern is shown among both the respondents and their parents.

When the family structure is considered, close to 70.0% of the respondents reported that they had lived in intact families until age 18. Blacks, however, tend to have a lower likelihood of staying in intact families until age 18 than non-Hispanic whites and Hispanics. In terms of religion, a slightly higher percentage of females reported that they were raised with religious affiliations than males (85.9 versus 81.3%). Among all respondents, higher percentages of Hispanics and blacks reported that they were raised with religious doctrines than non-Hispanic whites.

As far as the proximate determinants, females reported a greater average number of marriages than males (0.72 versus 0.62). There are also a higher percentage of females who had sterilization operations than males (18.2 versus 6.4%). Both the male and female respondents reported an average age at first sexual intercourse as 17. The racial and ethnic differences are also found regarding these proximate determinants. Specifically, Hispanics reported a lower average number of marriages (0.6) than non-Hispanic whites (0.7) and blacks (0.7). There is also a lower percentage of Hispanics who reported having ever conducted sterilization operations (11.2%) as compared to blacks (13.9%) and non-Hispanic whites (12.7%). Additionally, blacks reported a relatively earlier average age at first sexual intercourse (15.9) than whites (17.2) and Hispanics (17.3). The differentials by gender and race and ethnicity shown in the respondent's demographic and socioeconomic characteristics, family-background characteristics and the proximate determinants may have a significant influence on the respondent's cohabitation and fertility results.

In the next section of the chapter, I will apply statistical models to investigate how these factors mediate with cohabitation to influence male and female fertility, with a specific focus on the gender and racial and ethnic differences in the cohabitation and fertility correlation.

8.6.2 Poisson Regression Results

Table 8.3 shows the Poisson regression results examining the effects of variable *ever cohabited* and the interaction terms on CEB. Models 1, 3 and 5 focus on the effects of cohabitation on CEB after controlling for demographic and socioeconomic factors, family-background characteristics and the proximate determinants

Table 8.3 Poisson regression of CEB on ever cohabited variable, cohabitation interaction terms and other control variables by racial and ethnic group: U.S., 2002

	Whites		Hispanics		Blacks	
Variables	Model 1	Model 2	Model 3	Model 4	Model 5	Model 6
Cohabitation variable						
If ever cohabited (ref. = no)						
Yes	−0.12**	1.68***	0.20***	1.79***	0.46***	0.12
	(0.04)	(0.22)	(0.03)	(0.18)	(0.08)	(0.51)
Demographic factors						
Age	0.05***	0.07***	0.05***	0.07***	0.04***	0.05***
Gender (ref. = female)	−0.21***	−0.19*	−0.13**	−0.18**	−0.25***	−0.62***
Socioeconomic factors						
Highest degree R ever earned	−0.05***	−0.05***	−0.07***	−0.06***	−0.06**	−0.07***
Total combined family income	−0.01	0.01	−0.02**	−0.02**	−0.01	−0.02*
If R ever worked full time for 6+ months	0.41**	0.19	0.01	−0.04	0.28**	0.20*
Socialization factors						
Father's education	−0.02	−0.02	−0.02	−0.09***	−0.02	−0.14**
If raised up with a religious affiliation (ref. = no)	0.23**	0.23***	0.08	0.03	0.04	0.07
Proximate determinants						
Number of times R has been married	0.29***	0.72***	0.28***	0.93***	0.25***	0.53***
Age at first sexual intercourse	−0.02*	−0.02**	−0.02***	−0.03***	−0.04***	−0.09***
If R ever had sterilization operation	0.33***	0.09	0.18***	−0.01	0.30***	0.32***
Interaction terms						
Ever cohabited * gender		0.04		0.13		0.50***
		(0.09)		(0.08)		(0.15)

Table 8.3 (continued)

Variables	Whites: Model 1	Whites: Model 2	Hispanics: Model 3	Hispanics: Model 4	Blacks: Model 5	Blacks: Model 6
Ever cohabited * father's education		–		–		0.17**
						(0.06)
Ever cohabited * marriage		−0.49***		−0.76***		−0.32**
		(0.09)		(0.11)		(0.10)
Ever cohabited * age at 1st sex		–		–		0.06*
						(0.02)
Ever cohabited * sterilization operation		0.37***		0.26**		–
		(0.10)		(0.08)		
Constant	−1.48***	−2.36***	−0.35***	−1.28***	−0.30	0.31
N	5,397	5,397	2,104	2,104	1,817	1,817
Prob > F	0.0000	0.0000	0.0000	0.0000	0.0000	0.0000

"–"represents the regression coefficient being non-significant, thus, are not reported.

Sources: derived from NSFG Cycle 6 male and female datasets, 2002. Variables foreign born, metropolitan residence, mother's education and lived in intact family are dropped from the regression due to non-significant regression coefficients. Numbers in parentheses are standard errors associated with the regression coefficients.

for non-Hispanic whites, Hispanics and blacks, respectively. Models 2, 4, and 6 include the gender interaction term and the interaction effects of cohabitation with other relevant variables on CEB. I set the group of people who have never cohabited as the reference category in all models.

As the results show in models 1, 3 and 5, when all male and female respondents are analyzed and when other relevant factors are controlled, a cohabitation experience exhibits a positive effect on Hispanic and black CEBs but a negative influence on fertility of non-Hispanic whites. These results seem to partially support hypothesis 1 on a positive effect of cohabitation on fertility. After the interaction effects of cohabitation and other covariates (including gender) are taken into consideration in models 2, 4 and 6, the negative effect of cohabitation on fertility of non-Hispanic whites turns to be positive as well. Allison (1999) points out that whenever the interaction effect is significant in the regression model, the statistical significance of the main effect should not be a concern and researchers may need to focus on the model with significant interaction terms. In this case, since some of the interaction effects are significant in models 2, 4 and 6 (which will be discussed in the following paragraphs), the discussion of the results may need to be based on those models that contain the interaction terms. Thus, according to model 2, cohabitation has a positive and significant effect on fertility of non-Hispanic whites. Such a finding supports hypothesis 1 that cohabitation positively influences people's fertility.

When the gender interaction terms are considered, findings show that there is a significant fertility differential by gender due to cohabitation among blacks. Specifically, having ever cohabited increases a black female's CEB by 13% ($e^{0.12}$), whereas a black male's CEB by 86% ($e^{0.12+0.50}$). It suggests that cohabitation has a significantly stronger positive effect on black men's than on black women's fertility. This finding challenges hypothesis 2 that the cohabitation effect on fertility does not vary by gender. Such a gender difference, nevertheless, is not shown among non-Hispanic whites or Hispanics.

In addition to the fertility differentials by gender among blacks, it may also be observed that the cohabitation effect on black's fertility seems to be weaker than those on white's and Hispanic's fertility, considering the smaller regression coefficient for blacks as compared to those for whites and Hispanics. This finding weakens hypothesis 3 based on previous analyses that cohabitation has stronger positive effects on Hispanic's and black's fertility than on white's fertility. I suspect that the inconsistency between findings of this research and previous analyses may be due to the interaction terms added in this research. Indeed, the interaction effects between cohabitation and other relevant covariates are also more similar than different for non-Hispanic whites and Hispanics as compared to those for blacks. Results reveal that cohabitation has little effect on CEB through interacting with socioeconomic status of the respondent for all three racial and ethnic groups, which is against hypotheses 4 through 6. However, cohabitation shows significant influence on fertility of non-Hispanic whites and Hispanics through interacting with the respondent's marital experience and sterilization history. The interacting effects between cohabitation and age at first sexual initiation and father's education appear to be significant only on fertility of blacks (see models 2, 4 and 6 in Table 8.3).

These findings provide further evidence that the cohabitation effects on white's and Hispanic's fertility are more similar than different as compared to that on black's fertility, which challenges hypothesis 3. In the following paragraphs, I will explain in a greater detail how the interaction effects of cohabitation and other variables vary by racial and ethnic groups.

The regression coefficients of –0.49, –0.76 and –0.32 for the interaction between cohabitation and marriage in models 2, 4 and 6 inform us that the effect of cohabitation on childbearing decreases as the number of times the respondent has been married increasing. Specifically, the effect of cohabitation is given by 1.68–0.49*number of marriages for non-Hispanic whites. For Hispanics and blacks, the corresponding interaction functions are 1.79–0.76*number of marriages and 0.12–0.32*number of marriages, respectively. These functions support hypothesis 9 that the effect of cohabitation on fertility decreases with an increasing number of marriages. The above functions can be interpreted as follows: for blacks, cohabitation has a positive effect on fertility of those who have never been married. But such a positive effect turns to be negative for those who have a marriage experience. For non-Hispanic whites and Hispanics, the effect of cohabitation on fertility remains positive until the respondent marries over four times. The racial and ethnic differences again emerge in the cohabitation and fertility relationship. Non-Hispanic whites and Hispanics generally show a more similar than different pattern as compared to blacks. Non-Hispanic whites and Hispanics tend to be more "immune" to the marriage effect on fertility through mediating with cohabitation than blacks. The decreasing effect of cohabitation on fertility as the number of marriages increasing could be explained by the negative effects of marital disruptions that are associated with multiple marriages. Marital disruptions, along with insecurity and instability coming from dissolved relationships, decrease the likelihood of giving birth in a cohabitation union.

For non-Hispanic whites and Hispanics, the effect of cohabitation on fertility also varies by the respondent's sterilization history according to the interaction functions of 1.68+0.37*sterilization and 1.68+0.26*sterilization for non-Hispanic whites and for Hispanics, respectively. For both racial and ethnic groups, cohabitation shows a stronger positive effect on fertility of those who had sterilization operations than of those who had not done so. Such results are against hypothesis 10. This unexpected finding is probably because an individual who had a sterilization operation may have already reached his/her *desired* number of births. Thus, the person is more likely to have a higher fertility in a cohabitation union as compared to an individual who did not undergo a sterilization operation. Interestingly, however, the effect of cohabitation on blacks' CEB is independent of their sterilization history.

For blacks, in addition to the interaction effect of cohabitation and marriage, significant interaction effects are also found between cohabitation and *father's educational attainment* and the respondent's *age at first sexual intercourse*. These interaction effects are not shown among non-Hispanic whites and Hispanics. The function of 0.12+0.17*father's schooling in model 6 means that the positive effect of cohabitation on fertility increases with the level of parental education, which is against hypothesis 7. The cohabitation effect given by 0.12+0.06*age at first sex indicates that the fertility differences are more substantial among blacks with and without a cohabitation experience when age at first sexual initiation increases. This finding challenges hypothesis 9 that the cohabitation effect on fertility decreases as age at first sexual initiation increasing. I will discuss the mechanisms that have caused these results in the conclusion and discussion part.

On the whole, the results presented in Table 8.3 emphasize that cohabitation has a significantly positive association with male and female fertility. However, such an association ought to be explained by looking at the mediating effects of cohabitation with other factors rather than the main effect of cohabitation. I find a significantly higher level of male than female fertility among blacks owing to cohabitation. Black men appear to benefit more from cohabitation than black women. Such fertility differentials by gender are not shown among non-Hispanic whites and Hispanics. In general, the cohabitation effects on white's and Hispanic's fertility tend to be more similar than different as compared to the effect on black's fertility.

Beyond focusing on the effects of *ever cohabited* and the interaction terms on fertility, I find most control variables are influential as well. Among them, the religious variable, *if the respondent was raised with a religious affiliation*, deserves special attention because it shows significantly different effects on fertility across racial and ethnic groups. Being raised in a religious family significantly increases non-Hispanic whites' fertility but its effects on Hispanic and black fertility are trivial. This finding indicates that future research on causes of fertility differences across racial and ethnic groups could probably be directed to religious factors, such as religious affiliation and participation.

Table 8.4 shows the Poisson regression results based on analyzing samples without male respondents aged 25 and younger. As the results show, findings presented in Table 8.4 do not significantly challenge the conclusions drawn from analyzing all respondents although the magnitude of the cohabitation effect on fertility reduces.

I now turn to examine the effect of cohabitation experience on fertility by replacing the variable *ever cohabited* and the corresponding interaction terms by variable *cohabitation experience* and its related interaction terms. I decompose variable *cohabitation experience* into categories of "never cohabited," "cohabited only with spouses before marriage" and "cohabited with others that the respondent has never married." By doing this, "ever cohabited" that has been examined in earlier part of the analysis has been decomposed to two sub-categories as mentioned above. I set the "never cohabited" group as the reference category in all models in Table 8.5.

Compared to results shown in Table 8.3, though the cohabitation variables still show significant effects on fertility, some new findings emerge in Table 8.5. Before decomposition, only black men show a significantly higher level of fertility than black women due to cohabitation. After decomposition, male and female fertility differences caused by cohabitation are shown among non-Hispanic whites and Hispanics as well. To illustrate, as compared to respondents who had never cohabited, respondents who transformed their cohabitation relationships to marriages reported a significantly greater number of children. Also, male fertility seems to benefit more from transforming a cohabitation relationship to marriage than female fertility (see model 6 in Table 8.5). Such male and female fertility differentials

Table 8.4 Poisson regression of CEB on ever cohabited variable, cohabitation interaction terms and other control variables by racial and ethnic group: U.S. female samples and male samples 26 and over, 2002

	Whites		Hispanics		Blacks	
Variables	Model 1	Model 2	Model 3	Model 4	Model 5	Model 6
Cohabitation variable						
If ever cohabited (ref. = no)						
Yes	−0.09**	1.38***	0.15***	1.53***	0.37***	0.29
	(0.03)	(0.25)	(0.04)	(0.20)	(0.05)	(0.34)
Demographic factors						
Age	0.03***	0.06***	0.03***	0.05***	0.02***	0.03***
Gender (ref. = female)	−0.22***	−0.09	−0.08	−0.11	−0.16***	−0.45***
Socioeconomic factors						
Highest degree R ever earned	−0.05***	−0.05***	−0.07***	−0.06***	−0.07***	−0.07***
Total combined family income	−0.01	0.01	−0.02**	−0.02**	−0.02***	−0.03***
If R ever worked full time for 6+ months	0.35***	0.11	−0.11*	−0.12*	0.15*	0.12*
Family-background characteristics						
Father's education	−0.03	−0.02	−0.10***	−0.09***	0.01	−0.05
If raised up with a religious affiliation (ref. = no)	0.24**	0.23***	0.19	0.03	0.01	0.07
Proximate determinants						
Number of times R has been married	0.35***	0.67***	0.27***	0.80***	0.22***	0.47***
Age at first sexual intercourse	−0.01**	−0.02**	−0.03***	−0.03***	−0.04***	−0.07***
If R ever had sterilization operation	0.42***	0.12	0.34***	−0.01	0.44***	0.45***
Interaction terms						
Ever cohabited * gender		0.01		0.13		0.38***
		(0.10)		(0.09)		(0.13)
Ever cohabited * father's education		–		–		0.08**
						(0.05)
Ever cohabited * marriage		−0.45***		−0.64***		−0.30**
		(0.08)		(0.08)		(0.08)

Table 8.4 (continued)

	Whites		Hispanics		Blacks	
Variables	Model 1	Model 2	Model 3	Model 4	Model 5	Model 6
Ever cohabited* age at 1st sex		–		–		0.04* (0.02)
Ever cohabited* sterilization operation		0.34*** (0.09)		(0.10) (0.10)		–
Constant	–0.99***	–1.79***	0.34*	–0.57***	0.56***	0.78**
N	4,670	4,670	1,796	1,796	1,576	1,576
Prob > F	0.0000	0.0000	0.0000	0.0000	0.0000	0.0000

Sources: derived from NSFG Cycle 6 male and female datasets, 2002. Samples in this table are not weighted due to limited number of cases in certain strata after male respondents aged 25 and younger are dropped.

Table 8.5 Poisson regression of CEB on cohabitation variables, cohabitation interaction terms and other control variables by racial and ethnic group: U.S., 2002

Variables	Whites		Hispanics		Blacks	
	Model 1	Model 2	Model 3	Model 4	Model 5	Model 6
Cohabitation variables						
Cohabitation experience (ref. = never cohabited)	–	–	–	–	–	–
Only cohabited with prt(s) R married	−0.04	1.80***	0.18***	1.91***	0.31***	0.62
	(0.04)	(0.24)	(0.05)	(0.21)	(0.09)	(0.47)
Cohabited with partners R never married	−0.25***	1.70***	0.22***	1.63***	0.55***	0.20
	(0.05)	(0.27)	(0.05)	(0.23)	(0.08)	(0.59)
Demographic factors						
Age	0.05***	0.07***	0.05***	0.07***	0.04***	0.05***
Gender (ref. = female)	−0.19***	−0.19*	−0.13**	−0.17**	−0.29***	−0.61***
Socioeconomic factors						
Highest degree R ever earned	−0.05***	−0.06***	−0.07***	−0.06***	−0.06***	−0.07***
Total combined family income	−0.01	−0.01	−0.02**	−0.02**	−0.01	−0.02*
If R ever worked full time for 6+ months	0.43**	0.21***	0.01	−0.04	0.27*	0.20*
Socialization factors						
Father's education	−0.02	−0.02	−0.10***	−0.09***	−0.02	−0.14**
If raised up with a religious affiliation (ref. = no)	0.19*	0.23**	0.07	0.04	0.07	0.03
Proximate determinants						
Number of times R has been married	0.27***	0.72***	0.28***	0.92***	0.31***	0.53***
Age at first sexual intercourse	−0.02*	−0.03**	−0.02***	−0.03***	−0.04*	−0.09***
If R ever had sterilization operation	0.32***	0.07	0.19***	0.01	0.32***	0.34***
Interaction terms						
Cohabited only with spouses * gender		0.16*		0.22*		0.43*
		(0.10)		(0.10)		(0.18)
Cohabited with never married prt(s)* gender		−0.08		0.11		0.47**
		(0.12)		(0.09)		(0.16)

Table 8.5 (continued)

	Whites		Hispanics		Blacks	
Variables	Model 1	Model 2	Model 3	Model 4	Model 5	Model 6
Cohabited only with spouses * father's edu		–		–		0.19**
						(0.06)
Cohabited with never married prt(s) * father's edu		–		–		0.16**
						(0.06)
Cohabited only with spouses * marriage		−0.65***		−0.84***		−0.39***
		(0.09)		(0.12)		(0.10)
Cohabited with never married prt(s) * marriage		−0.38***		−0.71***		−0.19
		(0.10)		(0.14)		(0.11)
Cohabited only with spouses * age at 1st sex		–		–		0.04
						(0.03)
Cohabited with never married prt(s) * age at 1st sex		–		–		0.07**
						(0.03)
Cohabited only with spouses∗sterilization operation		0.31***		0.30**		–
		(0.09)		(0.09)		
Cohabited with never married prt(s)∗ sterilization Operation		0.38*		0.24*		–
		(0.18)		(0.12)		
Constant	−1.42***	−2.23***	−0.36***	−1.28***	−0.28	0.34
N	5,396	5,396	2,101	2,101	1,816	1,816
Prob > F	0.0000	0.0000	0.0000	0.0000	0.0000	0.0000

"–" represents non-significant regression coefficient which is not reported in the table.

Sources: derived from NSFG Cycle 6 male and female datasets, 2002. Variables foreign born, metropolitan residence, mother's education and lived in intact family are dropped from the models due to non-significant regression coefficients. Numbers in parentheses are standard errors associated with regression coefficients.

among non-Hispanic whites and Hispanics are not shown when comparing fertility of respondents who never cohabited and fertility of those who had not transformed their cohabitation relationships to marriages. These results suggest that for non-Hispanic whites and Hispanics, it may not be a cohabitation experience but a cohabitation outcome which had been converted to marriage that increases male fertility to a greater extent than female fertility. For blacks, however, the stronger positive effect of cohabitation on black male than female fertility is independent of their cohabitation outcome. In this sense, cohabitation may have different meanings in terms of childbearing for blacks as compared to non-Hispanic whites and Hispanics. One may argue that the fertility differentials by gender shown here may be caused by underreporting of births by men rather than converting a cohabitation experience to marriage since men are more likely to omit births that occur in non-marital unions than women. If the argument is the case, then the fertility differentials by gender shown in this research deserve further investigation.

As far as the effects of other covariates on fertility, the findings suggest that the associations between cohabitation and the respondent's parental education and sterilization history are not affected by decomposing the respondent's cohabitation experience. However, decomposition does cause significant fertility differentials caused by cohabitation through operating with the respondent's marital experience and age at first sexual initiation. As results in Table 8.3 indicate, the effect of cohabitation on fertility decreases if the respondent has had a marital experience. Findings in Table 8.5 further suggest that for non-Hispanic whites and Hispanics, the cohabitation effect on fertility is decreased to an even lower magnitude if the cohabitation relationship is converted to marriage. For blacks, the cohabitation effect on fertility only varies by marriage if the cohabitation relationship is transformed to a marriage relationship (see model 6). These findings again imply that cohabitation outcome rather than cohabitation may have played an important role in determining fertility results, especially for blacks. In terms of the interaction effects between cohabitation and age at first sex initiation, the results for non-Hispanic whites and Hispanics are consistent with results shown in Table 8.3. For blacks, however, the cohabitation effect on fertility turns to vary by age at first sex initiation only if the cohabitation experience has not been converted to a marital experience. In such a case, the cohabitation effect on fertility for blacks increases with age at first sexual initiation increases.

Table 8.6 provides the Poisson regression results without males aged 25 and younger. The results show that after younger men are left out of the analysis, a cohabitation partnership that has been converted to marriage appears to increase white men's fertility to an even greater magnitude relative to white women's fertility. Fertility differences among Hispanic men and women become non-significant; black male and female fertility differentials reduce but are still significant (see Table 8.6).

In addition to findings that are related to gender differences, the regression analysis excluding males aged 25 and younger also shows that for blacks, cohabitation no longer medicates with father's educational attainments to determine fertility. It suggests that paternal education may only influence blacks' childbearing behavior in

Table 8.6 Poisson regression of CEB on cohabitation variables, cohabitation interaction terms and other control variables by racial and ethnic group: U.S. female samples and male samples 26 and over, 2002

	Whites		Hispanics		Blacks	
Variables	Model 1	Model 2	Model 3	Model 4	Model 5	Model 6
Cohabitation variable						
Cohabitation experience (ref. = never cohabitated)	–	–	–	–	–	–
Only cohabitated with prt(s) R married	−0.03	1.48***	0.12**	1.43***	0.26***	0.24
	(0.03)	(0.18)	(0.04)	(0.22)	(0.06)	(0.41)
Cohabitated with partners R never married	−0.18***	1.65***	0.19***	1.67***	0.43***	0.27
	(0.04)	(0.20)	(0.05)	(0.25)	(0.05)	(0.37)
Demographic factors						
Age	0.03***	0.05***	0.03***	0.05***	0.02***	0.03***
Gender (ref. = female)	−0.20***	−0.23*	−0.09*	−0.11	−0.19***	−0.45***
Socioeconomic factors						
Highest degree R ever earned	−0.05***	−0.05***	−0.07***	−0.06***	−0.07***	−0.07***
Total combined family income	−0.01	−0.01	−0.02**	−0.02**	−0.02***	−0.03*
If R ever worked full time for 6+ months	0.36***	0.21***	−0.11*	−0.12**	−0.01	0.12
Family-background characteristics						
Father's education	−0.03*	−0.03	−0.10***	−0.09***	0.01	−0.05
If raised up with a religious affiliation (ref. = no)	0.22***	0.26**	0.18	0.12	0.02	−0.01
Proximate determinants						
Number of times R has been married	0.34***	0.76***	0.28***	0.80***	0.26***	0.47***
Age at first sexual intercourse	−0.02**	−0.02**	−0.03***	−0.03***	−0.04***	−0.07***
If R ever had sterilization operation	0.41***	0.18**	0.33***	0.17*	0.45***	0.46***

Table 8.6 (continued)

Variables	Whites		Hispanics		Blacks	
	Model 1	Model 2	Model 3	Model 4	Model 5	Model 6
Interaction terms						
Cohabited only with spouses *gender		0.23**		0.10		0.34*
		(0.08)		(0.11)		(0.15)
Cohabited with never married prt(s) * gender		−0.02		0.33		0.35**
		(0.09)		(0.11)		(0.13)
Cohabited only with spouses * father's edu		–		–		0.10
						(0.06)
Cohabited with never married prt(s) * father's edu		–		–		0.07
						(0.05)
Cohabited only with spouses * marriage		−0.65***		−0.70***		−0.32***
		(0.05)		(0.09)		(0.09)
Cohabited with never married prt(s) * marriage		−0.42***		−0.58***		−0.23**
		(0.05)		(0.08)		(0.08)
Cohabited only with spouses * age at 1st sex		–		–		0.05*
						(0.02)
Cohabited with never married prt(s) * age at 1st sex		–		–		0.04*
						(0.02)
Cohabited only with spouses*sterilization operation		0.30***		0.19		–
		(0.08)		(0.11)		
Cohabited with never married prt(s)* sterilization operation		0.32***		0.25*		–
		(0.09)		(0.12)		
Constant	−0.95***	−1.79***	0.32	−0.59***	0.58**	0.78**
N	4,669	4,669	1,793	1,793	1,575	1,575
Prob > F	0.0000	0.0000	0.0000	0.0000	0.0000	0.0000

Sources: derived from NSFG Cycle 6 male and female datasets, 2002. Samples in this table are not weighted due to a limited number of cases in certain strata after male respondents aged 25 and younger are dropped.
"–" represents non-significant regression coefficients which are not reported in the table.

younger ages. Moreover, the interaction effects between the cohabitation variables and marriage and age at first sexual initiation for blacks all become significant. These findings again show that blacks stand out when contrasting results with and without younger men after decomposing a cohabitation experience. Decomposition of a cohabitation experience is particularly necessary when the black sub-population is taken into consideration. Overall, findings based on examining samples excluding younger males do not significantly challenge the results drawn from analyzing all male and female samples.

8.7 Conclusion and Discussion

In this study, I have extended existing research in regard to the link between cohabitation and fertility by incorporating gender and race and ethnicity into the analysis. By analyzing the U.S. samples drawn from the NSFG surveys Cycle 6, I make a clear point that cohabitation positively influences male as well as female fertility, controlling for other factors. In fact, the positive effect of cohabitation on male fertility is significantly stronger than that on female fertility, especially among blacks. If a cohabitation experience is further decomposed to a cohabitation experience that has been converted to marriage and a cohabitation experience that has never been transformed to marriage, then male and female fertility differences owing to cohabitation emerge among non-Hispanic whites and Hispanics as well. Findings show that transforming a cohabitation partnership to marriage raises non-Hispanic white and Hispanic men's fertility to a greater level relative to fertility of their female counterparts. For blacks, the stronger positive effect of cohabitation on fertility remains even after decomposition. Thus, findings of this analysis generally support a stronger positive effect of cohabitation on male than on female fertility. Meanwhile, the results indicate that for non-Hispanic whites and Hispanics, the cohabitation outcome, that is, whether cohabitation has been converted to marriage, may play a more important role than cohabitation experience itself in differentiate male and female fertility.

A few additional questions arise here regarding the above findings. The first question concerns why men's fertility benefits more from cohabitation than women's, especially among blacks? A possible explanation is that cohabitation may operate as a "poor man's" alternative form of marriage, which has less demands on economic certainty and men acting as breadwinners of a household (Landale & Forste, 1991). Additionally, unlike marriage, cohabitation requires weaker economic underpinnings, which "provides fallback strategies for men whose careers are not established" for childbearing and rearing (Smock & Manning, 2004, p. 100). Since black men are often located at the end of the socioeconomic continuum in the U.S. society, cohabitation perhaps provides black males a more practical alternative form of marriage for childbearing relative to other racial and ethnic groups. Given women are usually not considered as breadwinners, the "alternative type of marriage" effect on fertility of black females may not be as significant as that on black males. Thus, fertility of black males benefits more from cohabitation than fertility of their female counterparts. This rationale may also be applied to other racial and ethnic groups, including non-Hispanic whites and Hispanics to explain why there is a stronger positive effect of cohabitation on male than on female fertility.

The second question that is closely related to the first one asks why fertility of Hispanic men does not gain as much benefit as fertility of black men from cohabitation considering Hispanics are as socioeconomically disadvantaged as blacks. I argue that different cultures and norms towards marriage, cohabitation and family formation among subpopulations may explain the racial and ethnic differences here. Prior research shows that similar to non-Hispanic whites, Hispanics tend to treat marriage as the "modal pattern" of childbearing (Musick, 2002, p. 917). Similar to whites, Hispanics are also more likely to be in a trial marriage type of cohabitation. Blacks, in contrast, tend to be in a substitute for marriage type of cohabitation (Casper & Sayer, 2000). The different attitudes and views towards cohabitation to a certain extent determine the childbearing patterns of cohabiters with various racial and ethnic backgrounds. Due to different culture and norms, Hispanics are probably more inclined to legitimate births that occur in cohabitation unions than blacks. This may explain why the fertility differentials by gender for Hispanics are shown after decomposing a cohabitation partnership. That is, a cohabitation partnership that has been converted to marriage raises Hispanic male fertility to a greater extent than female fertility. The same rationale can be used to explain why a cohabitation relationship that is converted to marriage raises non-Hispanic male fertility to a greater extent than female fertility. The findings suggest that in some cases, cultural factors could be more important causes of fertility variation across racial and ethnic groups than socioeconomic status when studying male and female fertility differentials.

The third related question concerns why cohabitation in general increases male fertility to a greater extent than female fertility. When I provide answers to the first question that why black male fertility benefits more from cohabitation than black female fertility, I have already pointed out the "poor men fall back strategy for childbearing" rationale that may explain the fertility differentials by gender. Recent research by Teachman (2003) offers another explanation to the third question. Teachman finds that women who have only cohabited with spouses do not experience a greater marital instability. In contrast, women who cohabited with partners other than their husbands exhibit a higher risk of marital disruption. Those women are therefore at a higher risk of marrying multiple times, which as my results show, diminishes the cohabitation effect on childbearing. If Teachman's finding can be used to explain the fertility differences by gender shown in this research, then a prerequisite needs to be met. That is, gender difference also exists in the link between cohabitation and marital disruption. Specifically, cohabiting only with spouses decreases the likelihood of men's marital instability to a greater extent as compared to women. If this prerequisite is met, then having cohabited only with spouses is able to increase male fertility to a greater extent than female fertility. Empirical analyses are warranted to verify whether the prerequisite can be met.

Besides the fertility differentials by gender explored in this research, the chapter also reveals racial and ethnic differences in the cohabitation and fertility relationship. Researchers have showed that cohabitation significantly increases black and Hispanic women's fertility; but it has a less significantly positive effect on white women's fertility (Brown, 2000; Leridon, 1990; Loomis & Landale, 1994; Musick, 2002). My findings show that when cohabitation interacts with family-background characteristics and the proximate determinants to influence fertility, non-Hispanic whites and Hispanics indeed share more similar than different patterns as compared to blacks. For instance, cohabitation shows stronger positive effects on white's and Hispanic's fertility than on black's fertility. In addition, the cohabitation effects on fertility of non-Hispanic whites and Hispanics depend on the same covariates, such as marriage and sterilization history of the respondent. For blacks, the cohabitation effect on fertility varies by a different group of covariates, including age at first sexual initiation and parental educational attainment. The similar than different fertility patterns due to cohabitation between non-Hispanic whites and Hispanics shown in this research is contradictory to findings of previous analyses that the cohabitation effects on black's and Hispanic's fertility are more similar than different as compared to whites. I argue that the inconsistency may be caused by including the interaction terms between cohabitation and other covariates which have not been incorporated in previous research. The racial and ethnic differences found in this research may be considered as a contribution to the existing literature, which highlights the importance of including the interaction effects in cohabitation and fertility studies.

Marriage is found to mediate with cohabitation to influence people's fertility for all three racial and ethnic groups. The effect of cohabitation on childbearing diminishes with the increasing number of marriages. For blacks, in particular, when marriage is taken into consideration, cohabitation shows a negative effect on black fertility. One of the previous studies by Manning on cohabiters' fertility shows that cohabiters with a marital history are more inclined to have planned births relative to those cohabiters who have never married (Manning, 2001). Although my research does not provide evidence supporting Manning's results, my findings are not opposing to Manning's study. Instead, my research results enrich the existing work by suggesting that cohabitation may operate with marriage in a positive direction when it comes to people's *desired* and planned fertility. Nevertheless, if people's *completed* fertility, such as CEB, is considered, cohabitation actually operates with marriage in a negative direction. Marital disruptions associated with multiple marriages decrease the odds of people giving birth in cohabitation unions. This interpretation falls in line with previous research on the negative association between marriage disruption and childbearing (Wildsmith & Raley, 2006). The racial and ethnic differences demonstrated in the interaction effects between cohabitation and marriage may result from differences in the role and meaning of marriage across subsamples.

It also worth to point out that highlighting marriage diminishes the effect of cohabitation on childbearing does not necessarily downplay the positive influence of marriage on fertility. As it can be seen in Tables 8.3 and 8.4, marriage increases people's fertility outcome even after a cohabitation experience is considered. Therefore, reinforcing marriage laws, including marriage education, incentives for marriage preparation, the reduction of the marriage tax penalty, and marriage support, which are proposed by researchers (Gardiner, Fishman, Nikolov, Glosser, & Laud, 2002) can still be considered as feasible strategies to increase fertility in low-fertility countries.

The family-background characteristic, *father's schooling*, is found to mediate with cohabitation only among blacks. The cohabitation effect rises with paternal educational attainments increasing. This finding is contradictory to what the prior literature states that cohabitation has a stronger positive effect on nonmarital childbearing among women of less parental investment (South, 1999). I am not sure how to interpret this discrepancy. One possible explanation of my finding could be that blacks with higher parental educational attainments enjoy a higher socioeconomic status, which allows them to afford a greater number of children as compared to those in a lower socioeconomic status in the same racial group.

In addition to the interaction effect between cohabitation and parental education, the results show that cohabitation has a stronger positive effect on fertility among blacks who initiated sexual activity at later ages relative to those who started sexual activity at younger ages. This is probably because earlier sexual initiation, as the prior literature suggests, is often associated with disadvantaged socioeconomic status, single-parent family background and segregated neighborhoods (Thornto, 1990). If this is the case, then blacks who started sexual intercourse at later ages are likely to be raised in relatively more socioeconomically advantaged families. Since blacks tend to remain in cohabitation unions for a longer period of time, blacks with higher socioeconomic status may be able to afford having a greater number of children while cohabiting. Thus, cohabitation shows a stronger positive effect on fertility of those blacks who initiated sexual activities in later ages. Age at first sexual initiation does not show significant interaction effects with cohabitation when influencing fertility for whites or Hispanics. This is probably due to little variation of ages at first sexual initiation among non-Hispanic white and Hispanic samples in this dataset.

In sum, this chapter explores the mechanism through which cohabitation affects fertility and how this mechanism varies by gender and across racial and ethnic groups. I clearly show that people's cohabitation experience influences their childbearing outcome through interacting with other relevant factors. Men's fertility in general benefits more from cohabitation than women's fertility. This "male advantage" phenomenon among non-Hispanic whites and Hispanics heavily depends on whether a cohabitation experience has been converted to marriage. Nevertheless, there is no such a restriction for blacks. These findings remind researchers to consider gender, racial and ethnic differences when studying cohabitation and fertility.

Previous research has highlighted a strong correlation between socioeconomic status and cohabitation in fertility. My results show that the demographic covariate (gender), family-background and the proximate determinants indeed have stronger interaction effects with cohabitation than socioeconomic factors to affect cohabiters' fertility results. These findings direct future research attention to non-socioeconomic factors when studying cohabitation.

Finally, I want to point out some limitations of the research in this chapter. First, I have not taken the duration of cohabitation into consideration. Researchers argue that the duration of the relationship is the key that distinguishes cohabitation from marriage (Briens & Joyner, 1988). As Manning (1995) states, the amount of time spent living together rather than having a cohabitation experience affects the timing of motherhood. Thus, considering the duration of cohabitation may help to disentangle the mediating effect between cohabitation and marriage on fertility. When racial and ethnic differences are taken into consideration, Hispanics and blacks usually stay in cohabitation unions for a longer period of time than non-Hispanic whites. The duration of cohabitation may influence the fertility outcomes of various racial and ethnic groups. Future work may control the duration of cohabitation to improve this current analysis. Second, I have not controlled for contextual and cultural factors such as cultural norms of subpopulations towards cohabitation and marriage and characteristics of the marriage market, which are found to affect cohabitation and childbearing behaviors (Jones, 2007). Future research may consider taking these factors into consideration. Moreover, I have very limited measures of socioeconomic status in this research which may have caused the interaction effects between cohabitation and socioeconomic variables being non-significant. Better measures of socioeconomic factors are warranted to examine how a variety of covariates and cohabitation come together to determine people's fertility results.

References

Allison, P. (1999). *Multiple regression: A primer* (1st ed.). Thousand Oaks, CA: Pine Forge Press.

Althaus, F. (1997). Children from disrupted families begin having sex, and children, at early age. *Family Planning Perspectives, 29*(5), 240–242.

Bachrach, C. A. (1987). Cohabitation and reproductive behavior in the U.S. *Demography, 24*(4), 623–637.

Bachrach, C., Hindin, M., & Thomson, E. (2000). The changing shape of ties that bind: An overview and synthesis. In L. Waite (Ed.), *The ties that bind: Perspective on marriage and cohabitation*. Hawthorne, NY: Aldine De Gruyer.

Bachu, A. (1999). *Trends in premarital childbearing*: 1930 *to* 1994. Washington, DC: U.S. Census Bureau.

Ballard, B. N. (2004). *Patterns of intended and actual fertility among sub-groups of foreign-born and native-born Latinas*. College Station, TX: Texas A&M University.

Berrington, A. & Diamond, D. (1999). Marital dissolution among the 1958 british birth cohort: The role and cohabitation. *Population Studies, 58*(1), 19–38.

Bianchi, S. M. & Robinson, J. (1997). What did you do today? Children's use of time, family composition and the acquisition of social capital. *Journal of Marriage and Family, 59*(2), 332–344.

Blanc, A. K. (1984). *The impact of changing family patterns on reproductive behavior: Nonmarital cohabitation and fertility in Norway*. Paper presented at the Population Association of America Annual Meetings, Minneapolis, MN.

Bloom, D. & Trussell, J. (1984). What are the determinants of delayed childbearing and permanent childlessness in the United States? *Demography, 21*(4), 591–611.

Briens, J. & Joyner, K. (1988). The ties that bind: Commitment and stability in the modern union. *American Sociological Review, 64*(3), 333–356.

Brown, S. L. (2000). Union transitions among cohabitors: The significance of relationship assessments and expectations. *Journal of Marriage and Family, 62*(3), 833–846.

Budig, M. J. (2003). Are women's employment and fertility histories interdependent? An examination of causal order using event history analysis. *Social Science Research, 32*(3), 376–401.

Bumpass, L. & Sweet, J. (1989). Children's experience in single-parent families: Implications of cohabitation and marital transitions. *Family Planning Perspectives, 21*(6), 256–260.

Caldwell, J. C. (1982). *Theories of fertility decline*. London: Academic Press.

Carlson, E. (1986). Couples without children: premarital cohabitation in France. In K. Davis (Ed.), *Contemporary marriage: Comparative perspectives on a changing institution*. New York: Russell Sage Foundation.

Casper, L. M. & Sayer, L. C. (2000). *Cohabitation transitions: Different attitudes and purposes, different path*. Paper presented at the Population Association of America, Los Angeles.

Chang, M. C., Freedman, R., & Sun, T. H. (1987). Trends in fertility, family size preferences, and family planning practices in Taiwan, 1961-85. *Studies in Family Planning, 18*(6), 320–337.

Cherlin, A. (1992). *Marriage, divorce, remarriage*. Cambridge, MA: Harvard University Press.

Clarkberg, M. (1999). The price of partnering: The role of economic well-being in young adults' first union experience. *Social Forces, 77*(3), 945–968.

Ellison, C., Echevarria, S., & Smith, B. (2005). Religion and abortion attitudes among U.S. hispanics: Findings from the 1990 latino national political survey. *Social Science Quarterly, 86*(1), 192–208.

Fields, J. & Casper, L. (2001). *America's families and living arrangements: Population characteristics*. Washington, DC: U.S. Census Bureau.

Gardiner, K., Fishman, M. E., Nikolov, P., Glosser, A., & Laud, S. (2002). *State policies to promote marriage: Final report*. Washington, DC: U.S. Department of Health and Human Services.

Goldstein, J. & Kenney, C. T. (2001). Marriage delayed or marriage foregone? New cohort forecasts of first marriage for U.S. women. *American Sociological Review, 66*(4), 506–519.

Jones, G. W. (2007). Delayed marriage and very low fertility in Pacific Asia. *Population and Development Review, 33*(3), 453–478.

Jurecki-Tiller, M. (2004). *The influence of religion on childbearing: Fertility, reproductive biology and belief in the church of Jesus Christ of latter-day saints*. Unpublished Dissertation, The State University of New York at Buffalo, Buffalo, NY.

Kamp Dush, C. M., Cohan, C., & Amato, P. R. (2003). The relationship between cohabitation and marital quality and stability: Change across cohorts. *Journal of Marriage and Family, 65*(3), 539–549.

Knodel, J., Chamratrithirong, A., & Debavalya, N. (1987). *Thailand's reproductive revolution: Rapid fertility decline in a third world setting*. Madison, WI: University of Wisconsin Press.

Landale, N. S. & Forste, R. (1991). Patterns of entry into cohabitation and marriage among mainland Puerto Rican women. *Demography, 28*(4), 587–607.

Lehrer, E. L. (1996). The role of the husband's religious affiliation in the economic and demographic behavior of families. *Journal for the Scientific Study of Religion, 35*(2), 145–155.

Leridon, H. (1990). Extra-marital cohabitation and fertility. *Population Studies, 44*(3), 469–487.

Loomis, L. S. & Landale, N. S. (1994). Nonmarital cohabitation and childbearing among black and white American women. *Journal of Marriage and Family, 56*(4), 191–200.

Manning, W. D. (1995). Cohabitation, marriage, and entry into motherhood. *Journal of Marriage and the Family, 57*(1), 191–200.

Manning, W. D. (2001). Childbearing in cohabiting unions: Racial and ethnic differences. *Family Planning Perspectives, 33*(5), 217–223.

McLanahan, S. & Bumpass, L. (1988). Intergenerational consequences of family disruption. *American Journal of Sociology, 94*(1), 130–152.

McLanahan, S. & Sandefur, G. D. (1994). *Growing up with a single parent*. Cambridge, MA: Harvard University Press.

Miller, B. C. & Heaton, T. B. (1991). Age at first sexual intercourse and the timing of marriage and childbirth. *Journal of Marriage and the Family, 53*(3), 719–732.

Mosher, W. D., Johnson, D. P., & Horn, M. C. (1986). Religion and fertility in the United States: The importance of marriage patterns and Hispanic origin. *Demography, 23*(3), 367–379.
Musick, K. (2002). Planned and unplanned childbearing among unmarried women. *Journal of Marriage and Family, 64*(4), 915–929.
Raley, R. K. (2001). Increasing fertility in cohabiting unions: Evidence for the second demographic transition in the United States? *Demography, 38*(1), 59–66.
Rendall, M. S., Joyner, K., Peters, H. E., Yang, F., Handcock, M. S., & Ryan, A. (2006). *A Bayesian approach to combining population and survey data for male fertility estimation*. Paper presented at the Annual Meetings of Population Association of America, Los Angeles.
Rindfuss, R. R., Morgan, P., & Swicegood, G. (1988). *First birth in America*. Los Angeles: University of California Press.
Rindfuss, R. R. & Vandenheuvel, A. (1990). Cohabitation: Precursor to marriage or an alternative to being single? *Population and Development Review, 16*(4), 703–726.
Sander, W. (1992). Catholicism and the economics of fertility. *Population Studies, 46*(3), 477–489.
Seltzer, J. A. (2004). Cohabitation in the United States and Britain: Demography, kinship, and the future. *Journal of Marriage and Family, 66*(4), 921–928.
Smock, P. J. & Manning, W. D. (2004). Living together unmarried in the United States: Demographic perspectives and implications for family policy. *Law & Policy, 26*(1), 87–116.
South, S. J. (1999). Historical changes and life course variation in the determinants of premarital childbearing. *Journal of Marriage and Family, 61*(3), 752–763.
Teachman, J. D. (2003). Premarital sex, premarital cohabitation, and the risk of subsequent marital dissolution among women. *Journal of Marriage and Family, 65*(2), 444–455.
Thomson, E., McLanahan, S. S., & Curtin, R. B. (1992). Family structure, gender, and parental socialization. *Journal of Marriage and Family, 54*(2), 368–378.
Thornto, A. (1990). The courtship process and adolescent sexuality. *Journal of Family Issues, 11*(3), 239–273.
Wildsmith, E. & Raley, R. K. (2006). Race-ethnic differences in nonmarital fertility: A focus on Mexican American women. *Journal of Marriage and Family, 68*(2), 491–508.

Chapter 9
Cultural Inheritance and Male and Female Fertility

In recent years, research interest is growing in the application of the cultural perspective to explain fertility variation. For instance, Susan Watkins (1991) has developed the diffusion theory of culture and cultural norms to understand the causes of the fertility transition in European countries from 1870 to 1960. She suggests that geographic diffusion of the innovation of fertility limitation within marriage was the key to fertility reduction in Europe. Since France was one of the most dominant areas of Europe, Watkins proposes that social pressures, reflected by the timing and extent of each province's integration into the French nation, was a main factor that has shaped marriage and childbearing patterns. She shows that the proportion of residents who spoke French was the best indicator of whether individuals were part of a national network. Joining that network has encouraged individuals to be responsive to national patterns of expectations about marriage and childbearing. Watkins' diffusion/cultural perspective has made a significant contribution to fertility theories by emphasizing the importance of culture and cultural norms as they influence fertility. The cultural perspective implies that cultural factors could affect fertility even in the absence of major structural changes at the societal level.

Following a similar vein, a few other fertility studies have also demonstrated the effects of culture on fertility at the *macro* level (Boling, 2008; Cornell, 1996; Murphy, 2003; Thomas, 1993). Recently, *Not by Genes Alone: How Culture Transformed Evolution*, by environmental scientist Peter Richerson and anthropologist Robert Boyd, has addressed the influence of culture, specifically, cultural inheritance on evolutionary outcome from a coevolutionary perspective at the *micro* level. Richerson and Boyd argue that cultural inheritance is analogous to genetic inheritance. During evolution, individuals who obtain cultural traits from parents are more likely to show resemblance between themselves (the offspring) and their parents. If the reproduction process can be viewed as part of the evolutionary process, then according to Richerson and Robert, cultural traits inherited from parents would result in more similar fertility outcome between offspring and parents. In a declining fertility regime, Richerson and Robert's argument seems to suggest that cultural inheritance from parents could be factor that prevents fertility decline. Such an argument echoes the implication drawn from Watkins' findings, that is, cultural norms

L. Zhang, *Male Fertility Patterns and Determinants*, The Springer Series on Demographic Methods and Population Analysis 27, DOI 10.1007/978-90-481-8939-7_9,

within the family system performed as a preventive factor of fertility reduction in Europe. This is because culture of fertility reduction coming from outside the family and village systems was an accelerator of fertility decline in European countries.

In this chapter, I use empirical data to test Richerson and Robert's theory of cultural inheritance in explaining male and female fertility. The research enriches existing fertility theories by incorporating the coevolutionary approach into the analytical scope. Additionally, the analysis addresses an important issue that the diffusion theory of culture has implied but not directly touched on, that is, whether cultural norms from inside the family are likely to be associated with higher fertility for both sexes. Before I move to the empirical analysis, I will first review culture and coevolutionary theories, which builds a theoretical link between cultural inheritance and fertility.

9.1 Theories and Hypotheses

At the beginning of the chapter, I have discussed the cultural tradition of studying fertility in demography. The importance of culture in determining evolutionary outcome, including reproductive outcome, has indeed been documented by the coevolutionary theory in anthropology as well. The coevolutionary approach argues that humans evolve via two interdependent inheritance systems: *genetic* and *cultural* (Durham, 1991; Lumsden & Wilson, 1981). Culture, as it affects human behavior, is considered on an equal status with genes because culture produces its own evolutionary dynamics and outcome that are not predicted by assumptions of natural selection working alone on genes (Rogers, 1988; Tinbergen, 1951). Here "culture" is defined as information that is socially transmitted between individuals (Cronk, 1995; Flinn, 1997; Richerson & Boyd, 2005). This definition is in contrast to culture defined as individuals learning the environment on their own and cultural information being obtained genetically.

According to anthropologists, there are two ways that culture is transmitted among generations during the evolutionary process: (1) from parents to offspring in a manner analogous to genes-this is referred to as unbiased or vertical transmission; (2) from non parental sources, such as teachers, peers and the media-this is referred to as biased or horizontal transmission (Cavalli-Sforza & Feldman, 1981). Richerson and Boyd (2005) argument explains why culture plays an important role in determining an evolutionary outcome. They contend that if children consistently adopt the traits of their parents in the absence of other forces, the composition of cultural traits within a population will not change over time. When it comes to fertility and reproduction, this argument makes intuitive sense because if one considers that to the extent that individuals act non parentally (produce few or no offspring), the cultural variants responsible for the reproductive restraint will be more likely to be removed from the population of parents and inherited by no one. If the reproductive culture is transmitted to the offspring without any biases, then the fertility outcome of parents and offspring would be expected to be the same.

In reality, both types of cultural inheritance are observed. When biased transmission is considered, Richerson and Boyd (2005, pp. 153–154) offer the example of teachers who are in a position to transmit ideas to large numbers of children. Teachers are also likely to hold views concerning reproduction that may differ, on average, from parents. This is because teachers themselves often have to delay marriage and reduce their own reproduction to be successful teachers. Depending on how much influence teachers have on children, the teachers' biased views towards reproduction may spread to their students. Teachers are just one of the many non parental sources of cultural influence that expose children to non parental ideas and lead to outcome other than those of their parents. Other sources of biased cultural traits include friends, priests, politicians, managers, entertainers and the media (Harris, 1998). In this way, biased cultural traits will increase the spread of cultural variant at a cost to an individual's reproductive success.

In sum, the coevolutionary theory discussed above suggests the importance of culture and cultural inheritance in shaping evolutionary outcome. According to the coevolutionary theory, the process of cultural inheritance can be considered as separate from that of genetic inheritance. Nevertheless, to a certain extent, the process of cultural inheritance is analogous to the process by which children inherit traits genetically from their parents. In this sense, coevolutionary theorists like Richerson and Boyd argue that the greater the degree of cultural transmission from parents to offspring, the more similar cultural inheritance will be to genetic adaptation. Consequently, there is a greater resemblance between parents and offspring regarding their evolutionary results.

Based on the preceding, I consider fertility outcome as part of evolutionary outcome and propose a *central hypothesis* regarding cultural traits and fertility transition as follows: the greater the extent that children have inherited cultural traits from parents, the more similar the fertility results of parents and offspring. It follows then that the offspring would maximize her individual reproductive success, slow down the fertility transition process and keep a high fertility. In other words, I anticipate a higher fertility level of offspring due to the influence of unbiased cultural traits. Thus, the hypothesis to be tested is operationalized as follows: individuals who have received more similar cultural traits from parents should have a greater number of children than those who have received less of those cultural traits. This is especially true in societies with a declining pattern of fertility. I test this hypothesis among both men and women.

9.2 Data, Variables and Methods

In order to test the central hypothesis proposed above, I use data from the 2002 wave of the National Survey of Family Growth (NSFG) Cycle 6 to conduct the analysis. The dependent variable is measured by the number of children ever born (CEB) to a male or female respondent. Similar to previous chapters, I obtain the CEB information based on the NSFG survey questions asking the female respondents "how many live births have you ever had?" and the male respondents "how many biological children have you ever had?" The analysis of this chapter contrasts the results based on including and excluding the male respondents aged 25 and younger, considering the issue of underreporting births by younger men.

The independent variable is *cultural inheritance*. There are a variety of cultural traits inherited from parents that could be analyzed. However, some of them may not be good measures of unbiased cultural traits although they show a strong parent-offspring correlation. This is because these cultural traits can be explained partially by genetics. For instance, political attitudes of the parents and the offspring are found to be related to each other. Nonetheless, political attitudes may not be considered as unbiased cultural traits since they show some genetic heritability (Alford, Funk, & Hibbing, 2005). Such measures are therefore avoided in the analysis since the focus here is the influence of unbiased cultural traits on fertility. In contrast to political attitudes, researchers find that some other cultural traits are less likely to be biased by genetics. One such trait is religious affiliation of the offspring; it has been found to be inherited from parents with little genetic transmission (Bouchard, McGue, Lykken, & Tellegen, 1999; Eaves, Martin, & Heath, 1990). Thus, such group affiliations are likely to be culturally derived (Alvard, 2003). Considering these matters and the availability of information in the NSFG Cycle 6 dataset for the respondent's religious affiliation, I decided to use the religious affiliation variable to capture the extent to which unbiased cultural traits are inherited from parents to offspring. This variable is chosen also because previous research has shown a strong association between religion and fertility (Bloom & Trussell, 1984; Jurecki-Tiller, 2004; McLanahan & Bumpass, 1988; Mosher, Johnson, & Horn, 1986; Rindfuss, Morgan, & Swicegood, 1988; Zhang, 2008). Prior research shows that religion is a very important factor that shapes people's fertility outcome. Thus, in this analysis, cultural inheritance is measured by the religious affiliation variable.

The religious affiliation variable that is used to measure *cultural inheritance* in this research is based on two questions in the NSFG Cycle 6 dataset. The first question asks the respondent about his/her present religious affiliation. The second question asks the respondent what his/her religious affiliation was when he/she was raised. I assume that the religion with which the respondent was raised should be the same as the religion of the respondent's parents. For example, if the respondent reported that he/she was raised as a Catholic, then I assume his/her parents were Catholics when he/she was growing up. Thus, if the respondent reported his/her current religious affiliation the same as that he/she was raised, I consider the respondent has inherited the same religious affiliation of his/her parents. In other words, the respondent has inherited unbiased cultural traits from his/her parents. Based on the two NSFG questions, I therefore generate a variable, *same religion*, to measure the extent to which the respondent has inherited unbiased cultural traits from his/her parents. I code the variable *same religion* as "1" if the respondent's current religious affiliation is the same as the one when he/she was growing up and "0" if otherwise. For those who have the *same religion* variable coded as "1" are considered as the respondents who inherited the same cultural traits (religion) from their parents, with the opposite for the respondents who are coded as "0".

When the respondent is asked his/her current religious affiliation or religious affiliation the respondent was raised, there are eight choices that could be chosen: (1) no religion; (2) Catholic; (3) Baptist/Southern Baptist; (4) Methodist, Lutheran, Presbyterian, Episcopalian; (5) Fundamental Protestant; (6) other Protestant denomination; (7) Protestant-no specific denomination; and (8) other non-Christian religion. For simplicity, in this research, for those who reported "no religion" for both religious questions are also coded as "1" for they are considered as having inherited the same cultural traits from their parents.

Besides the dependent and independent variables, I have also included four types of control variables in the analysis: demographic composition, socioeconomic status, family background characteristics and the proximate determinants. Demographic and socioeconomic factors are controlled because extensive research exists on the relationships between demographic and socioeconomic factors and fertility (Ballard, 2004; Ellison, Echevarria, & Smith, 2005; Freedman, Whelpton, & Smith, 1961; Singley & Landale, 1998). Thus, age, race and ethnicity, nativity, metropolitan residence and number of times the respondent has married are controlled as demographic factors. Education, total combined family income, and whether the respondent has ever worked full time for more than 6 months are used as measures of socioeconomic status. The family background characteristics are such as parental and maternal educational attainments and whether the respondent lived in an intact family until age 18. The proximate determinant measures are age at first sexual initiation and whether he/she had a sterilization operation.

Since the research is interested in examining how cultural inheritance influences male fertility as compared to female fertility, I also include a gender interaction term, which is generated by multiplying the *same religion* variable by the gender variable that is coded as "1" for males and "0" for females. Females are set as the reference category. If the gender interaction term is statistically significant, it indicates that cultural inheritance influences male and female fertility in significantly different manners. Descriptive information for all variables discussed above is presented in Tables 9.1 and 9.2.

In addition to descriptive analyses used in the research, the Poisson regression models are applied to estimate the effect of *same religion* on CEB, which is expressed as the following:

$$\mu_i = \exp\left(a + X_{1i}b_1 + X_{2i}b_2 + \ldots + X_{ki}b_k\right)$$

Where μ_i is the mean of the distribution, which is estimated from observed characteristics of the independent variables; a is the constant; b_i represents deviation from the mean of the omitted category, which is the reference group. The X variables are related to μ nonlinearly. In this case, μ_i is the expected number of children born to a respondent based on whether the respondent had inherited the same cultural traits (in this case the same religious affiliation) from his/her parents, the demographic and socioeconomic status of the respondent and so forth. All cases in regression models are weighted based on the final weights of each sample given by the NSFG.

Table 9.1 Descriptive statistics for CEB, same religion and control variables used in the analysis: U.S. 2002

	Male (all respondents)			Male (26 and over)			Female (all respondents)		
Variables	Mean (or %)	SD	N	Mean (or %)	SD	N	Mean (or %)	SD	N
Dependent variable									
CEB	1.2	0.04	4,117	1.5	0.05	2,622	1.3[a]	0.03	7,642
Independent variable									
Same religion			4,927			2,744			7,643
Yes	71.0			67.0			73.0		
No	29.0			33.0			27.0		
Other variables									
R's religious denomination when R was raised up			4,907			2,735			7,619
No religion	8.2			6.6			7.8		
Catholic	35.8			36.4			35.1		
Baptist/Southern Baptist	19.4			20.2			19.1		
Methodist, Lutheran, Presbyterian, Episcopal Arian	16.5			17.9			18.4		
Fundamental Protestant	4.5			4.4			5.9		
Other Protestant denomination	5.5			4.9			5.6		
Protestant-no specific denomination	3.1			2.5			2.8		
Other non-Christian religion	6.9			7.1			5.4		
R's present religious denomination			4,910			2,734			7,620
No religion	18.7			17.3			14.1		
Catholic	28.8			28.9			28.7		
Baptist/Southern Baptist	15.0			14.8			16.9		
Methodist, Lutheran, Presbyterian, Episcopal Arian	13.3			14.0			15.4		
Fundamental Protestant	4.7			5.1			6.1		
Other Protestant denomination	6.8			6.7			7.4		
Protestant-no specific denomination	5.2			5.1			5.5		
Other non-Christian religion	7.7			8.1			5.9		

Table 9.1 (continued)

Variables	Male (all respondents)			Male (26 and over)			Female (all respondents)		
	Mean (or %)	SD	N	Mean (or %)	SD	N	Mean (or %)	SD	N
Control variables									
Demographic factors									
Age	29.8	0.23	4,927	35.3	0.16	2,744	30.0	0.17	7,643
Race			4,927			2,744			7,643
Hispanic	16.7			16.2			14.8		
Non-Hispanic white	65.4			67.0			64.7		
Non-Hispanic black	11.9			10.9			14.0		
Non-Hispanic other	6.0			5.9			5.6		
Nativity-if foreign born			4,925			2,733			7,643
Native born	84.7			83.3			85.7		
Foreign born	15.3			16.7			14.3		
Number of times R has been married	0.6	0.02	4,927	0.9	0.02	2,744	0.7	0.02	7,643
Metropolitan residence			4,927			2,744			7,643
MSA, central city	48.0			48.4			49.0		
MSA, other	33.3			32.4			33.3		
Not MSA	18.6			19.2			17.7		
Socioeconomic factors									
Education			4,927			2,744			7,643
No diploma	22.9			15.6			21.2		
High school or less	31.5			33.5			28.3		
Some college/college	26.1			25.7			30.4		
University and above	19.5			25.3			20.1		
If R ever worked full time for 6+ months			4,925			2,742			7,636
Yes	79.1			96.7			74.1		
No	20.9			3.3			25.9		

Table 9.1 (continued)

Variables	Male (all respondents)			Male (26 and over)			Female (all respondents)		
	Mean (or %)	SD	N	Mean (or %)	SD	N	Mean (or %)	SD	N
Combined family income			4,927			2,744			7,643
Under $25,000	27.4			23.2			33.1		
$25,000–$49,999	33.3			35.4			30.3		
$50,000–$74,999	18.5			19.7			18.9		
$75,000 and over	20.8			21.8			17.7		
Proximate determinants									
Age at 1st sexual intercourse	17.0	0.08	4,108	17.4	0.1	2,612	17.3	0.06	6,785
If R ever had sterilization operation			4,925			2,742			7,643
Yes	6.4			9.8			18.2		
No	93.6			90.2			81.8		

Note: some sub-categories may not add up to 100% due to rounding.
[a]The CEB value for women who are 26 and over is 1.8 with a standard error of 0.04.
Sources: derived from NSFG Cycle 6 male and female datasets, 2002.

Table 9.2 Percentage distributions of male respondents' religious affiliations raised and current religious affiliations (%): U.S. 2002 (N = 4,902)

	Current religion								
Religion raised	(1)	(2)	(3)	(4)	(5)	(6)	(7)	(8)	Total
(1) No religion	5.9	0.4	0.3	0.4	0.2	0.3	0.2	0.5	8.2
(2) Catholic	4.3	26.9	0.6	1.2	0.5	0.7	1.0	0.9	35.8
(3) Baptist/Southern Baptist	2.7	0.5	13.2	0.7	0.7	0.5	0.5	0.5	19.4
(4) Methodist, Lutheran, Presbyterian, Episcopal Arian	2.3	0.9	0.7	10.5	0.3	0.4	0.5	0.8	16.5
(5) Fundamental Protestant	0.9	0.0	0.0	0.2	2.8	0.0	0.4	0.0	4.5
(6) Other Protestant denomination	0.7	0.0	0.1	0.0	0.2	4.3	0.0	0.0	5.5
(7) Protestant-no specific denomination	0.5	0.0	0.0	0.0	0.0	0.0	2.4	0.0	3.1
(8) Other non-Christian religion	1.3	0.0	0.0	0.2	0.0	0.4	0.0	4.9	7.0
Total	18.6	28.8	15.0	13.3	4.7	6.8	5.1	7.7	100.0

Sources: derived from NSFG Cycle 6 male dataset, 2002. All cases are weighted.

Considering the issue of underreporting births by younger men, the Poisson regression analysis is broken into two parts, which shows the effects of *same religion* on CEB with and without younger men aged 25 and younger, respectively. It is assumed that if the results based on the two parts of the analysis are similar, then underreporting of births by younger men is not a serious concern of the research.

9.3 Results

9.3.1 Descriptive Results

Table 9.1 presents the descriptive information for variables included in the analysis. On average, females reported a higher CEB value than males (1.3 versus 1.2). With respect to the independent variable, over 70% of the male and female respondents acknowledged that they had kept the same religious denominations. There is a slightly higher percentage of females claimed so than their male counterparts (73 versus 71%). After males 25 and younger are dropped from the analysis, the percentage of the respondents who kept the same religions declines to 67%. This is an interesting finding, which suggests that with age increasing, the likelihood of people keeping the same religious denominations as they were raised with decreases.

Data also show that before the respondents reached age 14, the majority of the male respondents claimed themselves as Catholics (35.8%), followed by Baptists/Southern Baptists (19.4%), and Methodists, Lutherans, Presbyterians or Episcopal Arians (16.5%). These are the major religious denominations that the majority of the male respondents were affiliated with when they were raised up. The percentage distributions of the female respondents who claimed religious affiliations before they reached age 14 are similar to those of males (35.1, 19.1 and 18.4% for the above religious denominations, respectively). The results show that eliminating the male respondents aged 25 and younger does not significantly change the pattern of such percentage distributions of the respondents.

As far as the respondents' present religious denominations are considered, the descriptive results show that the percentages of the respondents who claimed themselves as Catholics, Baptists/Southern Baptists decrease for both males and females. However, the percentages of respondents falling into most of the other religious groups increase for both sexes. Particularly, the percentages of the respondents with no religious affiliations show a dramatic increase. These results imply a secularization pattern over time in the United States. Meanwhile, other religious denominations other than Catholic and Baptist religions are also gaining more disciples.

Since the *same religion* variable is the key independent variable of the analysis and it is generated from two religious variables, the percentage distributions of the respondents on the two religious variables are also analyzed and are demonstrated in a detailed manner in Tables 9.2 and 9.3. The two tables cross tabulate the percentage distributions of the male and female respondents' religious affiliation raised and current religious affiliation, respectively. As both tables show, the majority of the male and female respondents reported the religious affiliations they were raised the same as their current religious affiliations, which indicates a high level of cultural inheritance. At the meantime, there is a small percentage of people who were converted from being non-religious to being affiliated with certain religions (2.3% for males and 2.7% for females). There is also a small percentage of the respondents who changed their religious affiliations from one to another. In contrast to those who have changed from being non-religious to being religious, there is a relatively higher percentage of respondents who have changed from being religious to being presently non-religious. Based on the data, 12.7% of the male respondents and 9.0%

Table 9.3 Percentage distributions of female respondents' religious affiliations raised and current religious affiliations (%): U.S. 2002 (N = 4,902)

	Current religion								
Religion raised	(1)	(2)	(3)	(4)	(5)	(6)	(7)	(8)	Total
(1) No religion	5.1	0.4	0.4	0.8	0.3	0.3	0.2	0.4	7.8
(2) Catholic	3.1	27.4	0.7	1.0	0.8	0.5	1.0	0.7	35.1
(3) Baptist/Southern Baptist	1.4	0.2	14.3	0.8	0.7	0.5	0.8	0.3	19.1
(4) Methodist, Lutheran, Presbyterian, Episcopal Arian	2.1	0.5	0.8	12.4	0.3	0.7	1.1	0.5	18.4
(5) Fundamental Protestant	0.8	0.0	0.4	0.0	4.1	0.2	0.3	0.0	5.9
(6) Other Protestant denomination	0.8	0.0	0.0	0.2	0.0	4.3	0.2	0.0	5.6
(7) Protestant-no specific denomination	0.4	0.2	0.0	0.0	0.0	0.0	1.9	0.0	2.8
(8) Other non-Christian religion	0.4	0.0	0.1	0.1	0.0	0.9	0.0	3.8	5.4
Total	14.1	28.7	16.9	15.4	6.1	7.4	5.5	5.9	100.0

Sources: derived from NSFG Cycle 6 female dataset, 2002. All cases are weighted.

of the female respondents reported that they have presently become non-religious though they were affiliated with certain religions when they were raised. This secularization pattern seems to be more popular among men than among women. If the conversions among various religious groups are considered, it may be observed that there is a general trend that Catholics tend to lose some disciples whereas other religious groups such as Methodist, Methodist, Lutheran, Presbyterian, Episcopal Arian and other non-specified religious groups have gained some disciples. Such a trend is similar for both males and females. In general, no significant gender differences are observed when comparing the cross tabulation results shown in Tables 9.2 and 9.3.

Since detailed discussions on the respondent's demographic and socioeconomic characteristics and the proximate determinant variables have been covered by previous chapters, this chapter will not provide much discussion on descriptive information of these variables. Readers may refer to the descriptive results presented in earlier chapters or information shown in Table 9.1 for information of these variables.

9.3.2 The Poisson Regression Results

The Poisson regression results analyzing the influence of cultural inheritance, measured by the variable *same religion* are shown in Table 9.4. The most important result in Table 9.4 is the significant and positive regression coefficients for the *same religion* variable. For all male and female respondents, the *same religion* variable has a Poisson regression coefficient of 0.08. This result means that inheriting the same religious doctrines from parents increases the respondent's CEB by 8% ($e^{(0.08)}$). This positive and significant effect is net of the effects of many other control variables. This finding implies that receiving unbiased cultural traits increases an individual's fitness, which in turn increases the level of fertility. Such a finding supports the central hypothesis drawn from the coevolutionary theory and implies that the argument of the coevolutionary theory can be used to explain fertility changes.

The second important finding of this research is that the positive effect of cultural inheritance, measured by *same religion*, on fertility does not vary by gender. this is because the gender interaction terms for the two sets of analyses are not significant. Such a finding can be interpreted as: on average, fertility of the male or female respondents who inherited the same religious doctrines from their parents is 8% higher than fertility of those who did not inherit the same religions from their parents. The result implies that cultural inheritance measured by religious variables does not appear to be a factor that differentiates male and female fertility.

Similar findings are shown after eliminating males aged 25 and younger. Results show that the magnitude of the coefficient for the *same religion* variable remains the same. It is also statistically significant. For other variables, the regression coefficients for age and gender variables have been reduced but the directions and significance stay the same. The regression coefficients for the rest of the variables are also consistent with the coefficients presented in the regression models that

Table 9.4 Poisson regression of CEB on same religion, gender and other variables: U.S., 2002

Variables	All respondents	All females and males 26 and over
Cultural inheritance variable		
Same religion	0.08***	0.08***
Interaction term		
Same religion * gender	−0.01	0.03
Demographic factors		
Age	0.05***	0.04***
Gender (ref.= female)	−0.30***	−0.21***
Race (ref. = White)		
Hispanic	0.31***	0.29***
Non-Hispanic black	0.27***	0.26***
Non-Hispanic other	0.23**	0.23**
Number of times R married	0.26***	0.24***
Socioeconomic factors		
Highest degree R ever earned	−0.05***	−0.06***
Total combined family income	−0.01*	−0.01*
If R ever worked full time for 6+ months	−0.01	−0.03
Family background characteristics		
Father's education	−0.04*	−0.03*
Mother's education	0.01	0.01
If R lived in an intact family from birth to age 18	0.01	0.02
Proximate determinants		
Age at first sexual intercourse	−0.02***	−0.02***
If ever used birth control methods	−0.33***	−0.25***
If R ever had sterilization operation	0.24***	0.29***
Constant	−0.49***	−0.12
N	9,664	8,402
Prob > F	0.0000	0.0000

Note: * p<0.05, **p<0.01, ***p<0.001, two-tailed test.
Sources: derived from NSFG Cycle 6 male and female datasets, 2002.

include all male and female respondents. These results suggest that the potential bias caused by underreporting of births by younger men may not be a serious concern of this research.

Besides the effect of the *same religion* variable on fertility, most of the control variables are found to be influential. Age and marriage have significantly positive effects on fertility. Hispanics, blacks and other racial groups show significantly higher levels of fertility than non-Hispanic whites. Education and family income are negatively associated with the respondent's fertility outcome. Among the family background characteristics, as expected, father's education shows a negative effect on fertility. Nevertheless, mother's education and living in an intact family until age 18 do not exhibit significant influence on CEB. The findings suggest that parental educational attainment is probably a better predictor of offspring's fertility than maternal educational attainment. The proximate determinants also demonstrate significant impacts on the respondent's CEB, net the effects of other variables.

9.4 Conclusion and Discussion

In this chapter, I have studied the effect of inheriting unbiased cultural traits, measured by inheriting same religious doctrines, on male and female fertility. With data on U.S. male and female samples, the findings show a strong association between unbiased cultural traits and fertility for both male and female respondents. That is, individuals who are affiliated with the same religions as their parents tend to have a greater number of children than individuals who reported different religious affiliations from those of their parents. Thus, cultural inheritance measured by inheriting same religious doctrines seems to be a factor that influences male fertility. But since there is no significant gender difference in the cultural inheritance and fertility relationship, cultural inheritance represented by inhering same religious doctrines does not appear to be a factor that differentiates male and female fertility. This finding somehow echoes the results shown in Chapter 7 that religious factors do not differentiate male and female fertility in the U.S.

Beyond the above finding on male and female fertility due to cultural inheritance, the findings of this research also have significant contributions to the existing demographic theories: First, the findings concur with Richerson and Boyd's (Richerson & Boyd, 2005) argument that *biased* cultural traits could be one of the possible underpinning mechanisms that have caused the fertility transition for both sexes. In demography, a number of theories have been proposed to account for fertility reduction. Most of those theories, however, emphasize the role of industrialization and modernization in providing an aggregate setting that influences fertility (Blake, 1973). For example, Mason (1997, p. 444) argues that social factors such as female labor force participation, increased education of women, and the secularization of society which "are presumed to be caused by industrialization and urbanization" are possible mechanisms that have resulted in the fertility transition. In contrast to the industrialization and modernization perspective, this research takes a coevolutionary perspective by looking at the level of cultural inheritance to explain fertility outcome. It shows that the extent to which cultural traits are inherited from parents can be another mechanism that regulates fertility changes. The rationale behind this mechanism is that offspring receiving more cultural information from non parental sources (biased cultural traits) indicates a decreased fitness, which is represented a lowered level of fertility. Though receiving cultural information from non parental sources may be considered as a result of industrialization and modernization, the coevolutionary theory provides an innovative perspective to account for the fertility transition.

The second contribution of this research is that the findings extend the applicability of the diffusion/cultural perspective from explaining fertility changes at the aggregate level to the individual level. In the existing literature, most empirical evidence supporting the diffusion/ cultural approach comes from the aggregate level analyses. By examining individual level data, this research indicates that the diffusion effect of culture on fertility not only makes sense at the macro level but also at the micro level. That is, once cultural traits from other sources are diffused to individuals, the evolutionary fitness decreases. This decreased fitness in turn leads to the fertility transition that is featured by having a fewer number of children.

The findings of this research also direct a possible approach to study fertility from an interdisciplinary perspective. Researchers often face the problem of reconciling different views and concepts when taking a multidisciplinary approach. When examining the influence of cultural traits on fertility outcome, a question arises from this research is that how the role of culture can be reconciled with evolutionary theories to explain fertility. Coevolutionary theory provides a possible solution. It argues for a central place for culture alongside genes. The coevolutionary theory views the influence of culture on evolutionary results as analogous to the influence of genes on evolutionary results. Thus, offspring inheriting more cultural traits from their parents is analogous to inheriting more genetic traits from their parents. As a consequence, those offspring demonstrate a high level of evolutionary fitness, represented by a high fertility. This coevolutionary thesis is supported by empirical findings of this research, which suggests a possible solution to apply a multidisciplinary perspective to investigate fertility.

In addition to the above aspects, the research of this chapter also resolves some discrepancies between the evolutionary theory and fertility results. For instance, according to the evolutionary theory, populations with the greatest wealth should have a greater number of offspring because holding more wealth indicates a greater level of evolutionary fitness. Demographers, however, have observed an opposite pattern. That is, a negative association exists between wealth and fertility: wealthy people in fact tend to have fewer children (Borg, 1989; Butz & Ward, 1979; Muller & Cohn, 1977; Poston, 2000; Thornto, 1978). Some have used the quality-quantity tradeoff hypothesis to reconcile this discrepancy (Lack, 1968). Such a hypothesis, nevertheless, is not supported by empirical evidence which shows that wealthy individuals can, in fact, easily increase fertility and poor individuals do not suffer reduced long-term fitness because of the greater number of presumably poorer quality offspring (Kaplan, Lancaster, Tucker, & Anderson, 2002). Instead of taking the quality-quantity approach, this research solves the discrepancy from a cultural perspective. The research demonstrates that biased cultural traits could lead to a lowered fertility. For those individuals with high socioeconomic status, they may have received more biased cultural traits (from school, work and so forth) than their poorer counterparts. Consequently, their contacts with non parental sources are greater and their fitness, shown here as fertility, is thus decreased. Put differently, the effect of increased exposure to non parental cultural information on fertility that is supported by empirical findings of this research plays a key role to resolve the inconsistency between evolutionary theory and demographic results.

Limitations of this research also need to be addressed here. First of all, the analysis of this research is purely based on the U.S. samples. This restricts the capability of the results being generalized to other subpopulations. Future research could extend the analysis to other social contexts to verify the association between cultural traits and the fertility transition as shown here. Moreover, only religious affiliation is used as the measure of unbiased cultural traits. Future research may use other measures to capture the influence of unbiased cultural traits on male and female fertility.

References

Alford, J., Funk, C., & Hibbing, J. (2005). Are political orientations genetically transmitted? *American Political Science Review, 99*, 153–167.

Alvard, M. S. (2003). The adaptive nature of culture. *Evolutionary Anthropology, 12*(3), 136–149.

Ballard, B. N. (2004). *Patterns of intended and actual fertility among sub-groups of foreign-born and native-born Latinas*. College Station, TX: Texas A&M University.

Blake, J. (1973). *Fertility control and the problem of voluntarism*. Paper presented at the Scientists and World Affairs, Proceedings of the Twenty-Second Pugwash Conference on Science and World Affairs, London.

Bloom, D. & Trussell, J. (1984). What are the determinants of delayed childbearing and permanent childlessness in the United States? *Demography, 21*(4), 591–611.

Boling, P. (2008). Demography, culture, and policy: Understanding Japan's low fertility. *Population and Development Review, 34*(2), 307–326.

Borg, M. O. M. (1989). The income-fertility relationship: Effect of the net price of a child. *Demography, 26*(2), 301–310.

Bouchard, T., McGue, M., Lykken, D., & Tellegen, A. (1999). Intrinsic and extrinsic religiousness: Genetic and environmental influences and personality correlates. *Twin Research, 2*(2), 88–98.

Butz, W. P. & Ward, M. P. (1979). Will US fertility remain low? A new economic interpretation. *Population and Development Review, 5*(4), 663–688.

Cavalli-Sforza, L. L. & Feldman, M. W. (1981). *Cultural transmission and evolution: A quantitative approach*. Princeton, NJ: Princeton University Press.

Cornell, L. L. (1996). Infanticide in early modern Japan? Demography, culture, and population growth. *Journal of Asian Studies, 5*(1), 22–29.

Cronk, L. (1995). Is there a role for culture in human behavioral ecology. *Ethology and Sociobiology, 16*(3), 181–205.

Durham, W. (1991). *Coevolution: Genes, culture, and human diversity*. Stanford, CA: Stanford University Press.

Eaves, L. J., Martin, N. G., & Heath, A. C. (1990). Religious affiliation in twins and their parents – testing a model of cultural inheritance. *Behavior Genetics, 20*, 1–22.

Ellison, C., Echevarria, S., & Smith, B. (2005). Religion and abortion attitudes among U.S. Hispanics: Findings from the 1990 Latino national political survey. *Social Science Quarterly, 86*(1), 192–208.

Flinn, M. V. (1997). Culture and the evolution of social learning. *Evolution And Human Behavior, 18*(1), 23–67.

Freedman, R., Whelpton, P. K., & Smith, J. W. (1961). Socio-economic factors in religious differentials in fertility. *American Sociological Review, 26*(4), 608–614.

Harris, J. (1998). *The nurture assumption: Why children turn out the way they do*. New York: Free Press.

Jurecki-Tiller, M. (2004). *The influence of religion on childbearing: Fertility, reproductive biology and belief in the church of Jesus Christ of latter-day saints*. Unpublished Dissertation, The State University of New York at Buffalo, Buffalo, NY.

Kaplan, H., Lancaster, J. B., Tucker, W. T., & Anderson, K. G. (2002). Evolutionary approach to below replacement fertility. *American Journal of Human Biology, 14*(2), 233–256.

Lack, D. L. (1968). *Ecological adaptations for breeding in birds*. London: Methuen Publishers.

Lumsden, C. J. & Wilson, E. O. (1981). *Genes, mind, and culture: The coevolutionary process*. Cambridge, MA: Harvard University Press.

Mason, K. O. (1997). Explaining fertility transitions. *Demography, 34*(4), 443–454.

McLanahan, S. & Bumpass, L. (1988). Intergenerational consequences of family disruption. *American Journal of Sociology, 94*(1), 130–152.

Mosher, W. D., Johnson, D. P., & Horn, M. C. (1986). Religion and fertility in the United States: The importance of marriage patterns and hispanic origin. *Demography, 23*(3), 367–379.

Muller, E. & Cohn, R. (1977). The relation of income to fertility decisions in Taiwan. *Economic Development and Cultural Change, 25*(2), 325–347.
Murphy, R. (2003). Fertility and distorted sex ratios in a rural Chinese county: Culture, state, and policy. *Population and Development Review, 29*(4), 595–626.
Poston, D. L. (2000). Social and economic development and the fertility transitions in Mainland China and Taiwan. *Population and Development Review, 26*(Supplement), 40–60.
Richerson, P. J. & Boyd, R. (2005). *Not by genes alone: How culture transformed human evolution*. Chicago: University of Chicago Press.
Rindfuss, R. R., Morgan, P., & Swicegood, G. (1988). *First birth in America*. Los Angeles: University of California Press.
Rogers, A. R. (1988). Does biology constrain culture. *American Anthropologist, 90*(4), 819–831.
Singley, S. G. & Landale, N. S. (1998). Incorporating origin and process in migration fertility frameworks: The case of Puerto Rican women. *Social Forces, 76*(4), 1437–1464.
Thomas, N. (1993). Economic security, culture and fertility: A reply to Cleland. *Population Studies, 47*(2), 353–359.
Thornto, A. (1978). The relationship between fertility and income, relative income, and expected well-being. In J. Simon (Ed.), *Research in population economics* (Vol. I). Greenwich, CT: JAI Press.
Tinbergen, N. (1951). *The study of instinct*. Oxford: Clarendon Press.
Watkins, S. C. (1991). *From Provinces into Nations: Demographic integration in Western Europe*, 1870–1960. Princeton, NJ: Princeton University Press.
Zhang, L. (2008). Religious affiliation, religiosity, and male and female fertility. *Demographic Research, 18*(8), 233–262.

Chapter 10
Conclusion

Demographic and sociological studies of fertility have long been focusing on studying females and male fertility remains overlooked in the literature. In this book, I have attempted to address this void by taking a gendered perspective to compare and contrast male and female fertility rates at the aggregate level and their determinants at the individual level. The primary goal of this book was to show the manner in which male fertility distinguishes itself from female fertility and the capability of existing fertility theories in explaining male fertility. This exercise aimed to improve our understanding of male fertility patterns and determinants and to provide evidence which helps to construct fertility theories of men.

I began the book by providing a synthetic review of prior literature on men's fertility and related issues. The topics reviewed include comparative studies of male and female fertility, men's participation in fertility decision-making and family planning, male fertility modeling and men's life cycle events that are related to fertility. I pointed out the strengths and weaknesses of these studies and highlighted how this current research may improve the existing literature on male fertility. Chapter 3 introduced data and methods used in this book and addressed the issue of underreporting births by younger men and how this issue was handled in this research.

Chapters 4 and 5 started to examine male and female fertility empirically at the aggregate level. The total fertility rate (TFR) and the age-specific fertility rate (ASFR) were used as the major measures of fertility in these two chapters. Chapter 4 studied male and female fertility dynamics in 43 countries and places during 1990–1998; Chapter 5 focused on a specific locale-Taiwan and examined the changing patterns of fertility for males and females since 1975–2004. The United Nations *Demographic Yearbooks* and the *Taiwan-Fukein Demographic Fact Books* were major data sources used to conduct the analysis in Chapters 4 and 5, respectively.

Chapters 6 through 9 shifted the research interest to investigating male and female fertility determinants at the individual level. I employed the National Survey of Family Growth (NSFG) Cycle 6 database in the research and moved beyond the descriptive to the multivariate realm. By examining the U.S. samples, the book revealed how a variety of demographic, socioeconomic, religious and

L. Zhang, *Male Fertility Patterns and Determinants*, The Springer Series on Demographic Methods and Population Analysis 27, DOI 10.1007/978-90-481-8939-7_10,

cultural factors affect male and female fertility results. The findings also pointed out the factors that influence men's and women's fertility results differently. In the following subsections, I highlight the key findings of the book.

10.1 Summary of Findings

10.1.1 Male and Female Fertility Differentials in Rates

One of the most significant findings I have showed in this book is that male and female fertility patterns measured by rates (TFRs and ASFRs) are not identical. Based on examining the TFRs for men and women during the 1990–1998 period in 43 countries and places, it has been found that male and female TFRs tend to be similar in countries with TFR values lower than 2,200 where female fertility appears to be higher than male fertility. In contrast, male and female fertility appear to be more dissimilar rather than similar in countries and places where both male and female TFRs are above 2,200, with male fertility being higher than female fertility. Based on the findings, I proposed that the *replacement level of fertility* may be a critical point that differentiates male and female total fertility patterns at the aggregate level.

This assumption was corroborated by findings drawn from Chapter 5 that studied male and female fertility in Taiwan during 1975–2004. The results showed that male fertility in Taiwan used to be higher than female fertility before the TFR had reached the replacement level. In the late 1980s, male and female fertility began to have a crossover when both male and female fertility reached the *replacement level.* Afterwards, female fertility began to be higher than that of males. These results echoed findings presented in Chapter 4.

Several explanations were proposed in the book to address why the replacement level of fertility serves as a critical point that defines the changing patterns of male and female fertility. Those explanations were linked to issues, such as immigration and outmigration, mortality differentials by sex, and mate availability caused by unbalanced sex ratio at birth in some Asian regions.

Beyond the total fertility differentials by sex revealed by Chapters 4 and 5, the results of this book also demonstrated the age-specific fertility differentials by sex. The age group 30–34 has been shown in this study to be the threshold defining the male and female age-specific fertility correlations. Female fertility has a higher rate than male fertility before a population reaches such an age group. Afterwards, males begin to have a higher fertility than females. These results, coupled with Paget and Timaeus (1994) findings, suggested that the threshold effect of age group 30–34 does not seem to vary over time with the changing level of total fertility. In addition, the research showed that the male and female fertility differentials among age groups 45 and over are more significant in lower fertility countries (TFR<2,200). The greater age-specific fertility differentials by sex in countries with lower total fertility rates implied that the male and female age-specific fertility differentials may interact with the level of total fertility. I therefore concluded that in future, with total fertility declining, the age-specific fertility differentials by sex for age groups 45 and over would become even greater.

The results drawn from the analysis of Taiwanese fertility further exhibited that the age-specific fertility differentials by sex also vary by people's educational attainment. This research showed that education has a stronger negative effect on female than on male fertility for age group 15–19. The effect of education in differentiating male and female fertility seems to be trivial for age group 20–24. Then for age groups 25–40, the depressing effect of education on male fertility becomes stronger as compared to its effect on female fertility. Conventional demography has focused a great deal on the importance of educational attainment on deterring female fertility. My analysis highlighted that at the aggregate level, education can indeed deter male fertility to an even greater extent than female fertility at certain ages.

According the above findings, I drew the conclusions that male and female fertility in rates at the aggregate level are non-identical and the correlation between male and female fertility changes over time. In future, with a declining pattern of fertility, male and female total fertility differentials will shrink with female fertility being slightly higher than male fertility. Nevertheless, the male and female age-specific fertility differentials will persist. Given that the male and female age-specific fertility differentials exist mainly in younger (under 25) and more mature age groups (above 45), it would be far more important to take male fertility into consideration when studying human fertility in countries that are largely represented by young or mature populations.

10.1.2 Male and Female Fertility Differentials in Determinants

In addition to the male and female fertility differentials in rates, the book has also demonstrated the male and female fertility differentials in determinants. When studying fertility in Taiwan in Chapter 4, I have investigated the capability of fertility theories based on females in explaining male fertility variation. My estimations showed that although fertility determinants at the aggregate level impact men's and women's fertility similarly, models combining those fertility determinants are more powerful when explaining female than male fertility. Thus, there must be some factors that drive men's fertility outcome being different from that of women.

In order to explore those factors, I conducted individual level analyses in Chapters 6 through 9 and detailed the influence of demographic, socioeconomic, religious, cohabitation and cultural factors on both male and female fertility. Based on research done in this book, almost all variables studied are important covariates and work to shape fertility results for both males and females. Though most factors contribute in the same way to male and female fertility results, some variables have been found to have significantly different impacts on male than on female fertility.

Chapter 6 found that demographic and socioeconomic factors have significant impacts on male and female fertility. Most factors work in the way as the theories expect. However, some demographic and socioeconomic factors affect men's and women's fertility results in significantly different manners. When all male and female samples are included in the analysis, controlling for other factors, age, marriage and Hispanic origin increase men's fertility to a greater extent as compared to women's fertility. Family income increases male fertility but decreases female fertility. In addition, labor force participation shows a much stronger positive effect on male than on female fertility. These facts have long been ignored in demographic and sociological studies of fertility. The chapter offered explanations for why the differential effects have taken place. Most of the explanations are linked to gender roles, biological constraints and cultural norms, which accounts for the fertility differences by gender.

Chapter 7 examined the effects of religion and religiosity on male and female fertility. The results revealed that religion and religiosity are important factors that determine people's fertility results. Although the fertility differentials among various religious groups in the U.S. are shrinking, religiosity appears to have strong influence on religious people's fertility. The strength of religious beliefs is shown to be a better predictor of fertility than frequency of religious participation for both men and women. By analyzing the U.S. samples, the results suggested that religion and religiosity do not tend to be factors that differentiate men's and women's fertility results.

Through evaluating the influence of cohabitation on fertility, findings of Chapter 8 showed that having a cohabitation experience increases both male and female fertility, with cohabitation showing a significantly stronger positive effect on male than on female fertility. Such fertility differentials by gender due to cohabitation are especially significant among blacks. The chapter raised questions such as why men's fertility benefits more from cohabitation than women's fertility and why Hispanic male fertility does not gain as much benefit as black male fertility from cohabitation. I argued that cohabitation may offer men a fallback strategy for childbearing and rearing, especially for poor black men, since the cohabitation union has less demands on economic certainty. That is probably why male fertility benefits more from cohabitation than female fertility. I also contended that though Hispanic men and black men have a similar socioeconomic status, different cultural norms may have shaped Hispanic men's fertility outcome being more similar to that of white men when the influence of cohabitation on fertility is considered. The chapter also found that some factors, such as marriage, father's schooling, and age at first sexual initiation interact with cohabitation when affecting fertility. Marriage diminishes the effect of cohabitation on both male and female fertility. For blacks, the cohabitation effect rises with paternal educational attainment increasing. In addition, cohabitation has a stronger positive effect on fertility among blacks who initiated sexual activities at later ages relative to those who started sexual activity at younger ages.

Chapter 9 investigated the influence of cultural factors on fertility. It demonstrated that for both men and women, inheriting unbiased cultural traits, measured by inheriting same religious beliefs, from parents does promote both male and female fertility. The finding proved the capability of the coevolutionary theory in explaining male fertility changes. The exercise also contributed to the existing demographic theories in a number of ways. For instance, the findings extended the applicability of the diffusion/cultural perspective for explaining fertility variation at the aggregate level to the individual level. It also directed a possible approach to study fertility from an interdisciplinary perspective.

Overall, men's fertility outcome has been proved to be influenced by most of fertility determinants studied in a similar way as women's fertility. However, there are some demographic, socioeconomic and union formation factors play significantly different roles in shaping men's and women's fertility outcomes. These facts would not have been discovered if the research of this book was not conducted. The findings help to improve existing demographic theories on fertility when both genders are brought into the scope of fertility research.

10.2 Implications

Findings of this book with regard to the male and female fertility differentials contain important implications not only for theoretical framework constructing but also for family planning policy making. In terms of the theoretical framework, it appears evident that at the aggregate level, fertility theories based on females are not sufficiently satisfactory explanations for male fertility variation. Equal apparent is that there are significant and important differences in the manner in which fertility determinants impact male and female fertility outcomes. These findings suggest that the existing fertility theories based on females may be applicable to men; but certain modifications are warranted. The book suggests the dimensions of the modifications.

Additionally, conventional demographic transition theory has generally focused on the role of socioeconomic change as a major factor that influences fertility. The importance of cultural factors has been largely ignored. The exercise done by this research implied that cultural factors may have important explanatory significance for both male and female fertility changes, which can be largely independent of the level of socioeconomic development.

Because fertility patterns and outcome directly reflect the goals and effectiveness of family planning programs in various countries, findings of this research also have important policy implications. Marriage in this research has been shown to be a stronger push factor for an individual man's fertility than for a woman's fertility. In Taiwan, delayed marriage was also found to reduce male fertility to a greater extent than female fertility. These findings should remind family planning policy makers in high fertility countries to encourage later marriage, particularly for men. Providing education loans to encourage people, especially males to pursue higher education in order to delay age at marriage could be an effective strategy to lower fertility. In low fertility countries, on the other hand, offering special welfare as incentives to people to encourage earlier marriage, particularly for men, may well increase the fertility rate. Cohabitation has been found to have a stronger positive effect on male than on female fertility. This finding suggests that as an alternative form of marriage, the increasing number of cohabitation union in low fertility countries may deter the rapid declining rate of fertility.

The much stronger positive effect of labor force participation on men's than on women's fertility suggests the particular importance of offering job opportunities for men. This could be a possible solution for low fertility countries to increase the fertility of men. Since some implications discussed here emphasize offering particular family planning policies for men, policy makers may face the dilemma of gender equality and regulating fertility. They need to balance out these two and find suitable solutions in order to manage people's childbearing behavior.

10.3 Underreporting Births by Younger Men

The quality of male fertility has always been a concern of researchers when studying male fertility. As stated earlier, this is because females are more directly involved in fertility-related events. Their reports on fertility are believed to be more reliable than those of men. In the literature review part, I have included some discussions on the reliability of male fertility data showed in prior literature. Most studies did suggest that men tend to underreport the number of children born to them, especially children born outside of marriage and from previous unions (see discussions in previous chapters). The problem of underreporting births in the 2002 NSFG dataset that used in this research has indeed been pointed out by Rendall and associates (Rendall et al., 2006).

Considering the issue of underreporting births by men and the potential biases that this issue may bring to the research results, I have developed a strategy which broke the samples into two subgroups. The first subgroup contained all male and female samples and the second subgroup excluded males aged 25 and younger. The reason for doing so was that underreporting births often occurs among men at younger ages. Contrasting results including and excluding this group of younger men should, to a certain extent, exhibit the influence of underreporting births by men. According to the average age at first marriage for American men, I set age 25 as the threshold for dividing the subgroups. I would like to make it clear that my intention for developing this strategy was to evaluate the influence of underreporting births by younger men on the study results, but not to directly evaluate the reliability of male fertility data presented in the NSFG Cycle 6.

My results showed that, in general, findings based on analyzing all respondents and respondents that exclude men aged 25 and younger were consistent with one another except for the differences that lied in the effects of age, income, labor force participation and cohabitation on male and female fertility (see the discussions in Chapters 6, 7, 8 and 9). These results suggested that underreporting births by younger men in the NSFG dataset does influence the research results in some aspects. It reminds researchers who use the NSFG Cycle 6 data to study male fertility with caution. I admit that the strategy applied in this research which eliminates males aged 25 and younger is not able to fully remove the biases that underreporting births may bring to the results. There is certainly a great deal of work remaining in terms of evaluating the quality of male fertility reports.

10.4 Future Prospects

Though this book is among the first to provide a relatively comprehensive assessment of male fertility, the research has several limitations that need to be addressed. First, my interpretations of male fertility determinants are, to a certain extent, hindered by the information provided by the 2002 NSFG dataset. This is because questions about births of men in the NSFG Cycle 6 were not directly designed to study male fertility. Thus, measures of male fertility are limited. As mentioned earlier, the reliability of male fertility data has not been systematically examined and reported either, which requires researchers using this dataset to study male fertility with caution. For independent variables, due to data constraints, some male fertility determinants had to be represented by proxies of those measures. For instance, there were incomplete data about the proximate determinants of male fertility, such as men's contraceptive use and age at biological maturation. Therefore, the sterilization variable and age at first sex initiation variable were used as proxies of those two proximate determinants. In terms of the dependent variable, CEB, it is considered as a representation of completed fertility. It demands the independent variables to represent the features of the respondent before the birth event occurs. Due to limited data, some of the independent variables drawn from the NSFG data were unable to capture such features and thus were only considered as proxies of the ideal measures. For example, the measures of economic determinant of fertility and total combined family income in 2001, obviously occurred after the event of birth. I offer these caveats because the data are not perfect to study male fertility, but I believe that the findings, despite the shortcomings, are robust and informative.

Further, when selecting fertility determinants that need to be included in the research, I intended to focus the analysis on demographic, socioeconomic, union formation (cohabitation), religious and cultural factors. While the book did cover a range of variables under those rubrics, I recognize that there are some others that come under those headings but have not been included in the research. Those factors are such as sex education, number of children born to the mother, menarche or the indicator of men's biological maturation. They have been shown to have significant influence on fertility behavior in prior literature (Aneshensel, Fielder, & Becerra, 1989; Ballard, 2004; McKibben, 2003; Singley & Landale, 1998). Past studies have also provided evidence that both structural and individual characteristics shape the changing patterns of fertility (Mason, 1997; Poston & Dudley, 2000; Watkins, 1986). In my research on male and female fertility determinants, I was not able to conduct analyses which incorporate aggregate level factors into the estimation since data from the NSFG are restricted to the individual level. Additionally, the effects of fertility determinants shown in my results were all direct effects. The indirect effects of these factors on male fertility have not been taken into consideration. Longitudinal analyses of how demographic, socioeconomic and other factors shape male and female fertility have not been conducted. In future, I expect that broader and more informative conceptual frameworks will emerge as researchers carry on this line of inquiry. I also hope that appropriate data sets will enable future work to examine the more elaborate span of covariates in their multivariate effects on male and female fertility, which will enrich findings shown in this book and construct male fertility theories in a more comprehensive manner.

Besides these limitations, this research has also raised some additional issues to be pursued in future work. For instance, I have provided several explanations to account for male and female fertility differences in rates. For instance, I offered the explanation from the mate availability perspective due to unbalanced sex ratio at births to explain male and female fertility differentials. I also proposed that the male and female fertility differentials could be due to immigration and emigration and the mortality differentials by sex. Those explanations, however, remained to be proposals and they need to be tested by future research.

A gendered perspective has been taken to examine male fertility. Methodologically, the ratios of male and female TFRs and ASFRs as well as the gender interaction terms were included in the analyses to study fertility by sex. However, the models in this research should still be considered as one-sex models. This is because men's and women's fertility determinants have not been incorporated in the same models simultaneously. Future research may consider constructing two-sex fertility models to explore the fertility determinants for both sexes.

The fertility models presented in this research could also be improved by adding the characteristics of the respondent's spouse(s) or partner(s) since their characteristics influence fertility of the respondent. Failing to include their characteristics in this research is largely due to the fact that male and female respondents in the NSFG were not husbands and wives living in the same households. In contrast to the NSFG Cycle 6 surveys, the Demographic and Health Surveys (DHS) and the Mexican Migration Project (MMP) both contain fertility information for husbands and wives. Relying on fertility information of those data sets to incorporate husband's and wife's characteristics, such as both their ages, racial compositions, and sexual histories into regression models would help to construct the two-sex fertility models.

It has been pointed out that together with lowest-low fertility, unbalanced sex ratios at birth, and the demography of gay males and lesbians, male fertility and men's influence on childbearing decision-making have become emerging issues of population studies in recent years (Poston, Baumle, & Micklin, 2005). This book has revealed male fertility patterns and determinants in diverse societies. Future advances in male fertility data collection arising from the large-scale national surveys and improvements in statistical techniques would permitted more refined studies of male fertility. Both quantitative and qualitative studies are warranted to carry on research on this important topic.

References

Aneshensel, C. S., Fielder, E. P., & Becerra, R. M. (1989). Fertility and fertility-related behavior among Mexican American and non-Hispanic white female adolescents. *Journal of Health and Social Behavior, 30*(1), 56–76.

Ballard, B. N. (2004). *Patterns of intended and actual fertility among sub-groups of foreign-born and native-born Latinas*. College Station, TX: Texas A&M University.
Mason, K. O. (1997). Explaining fertility transitions. *Demography, 34*, 443–454.
McKibben, S. L. (2003). *The social construction of adulthood: Menarche and motherhood*. Unpublished Dissertation, Texas A&M University, College Station, TX.
Paget, W. J. & Timaeus, I. M. (1994). A relational Gompertz model of male fertility: Development and assessment. *Population Studies, 48*(2), 333–340.
Poston, D. L., Baumle, A. K., & Micklin, M. (2005) Epilogue: Needed research in demography. In D. L. Poston, M. Micklin (Eds.), *Handbook of population* (pp. 853–883). New York: Springer Publishers.
Poston, J. & Dudley, L. (2000). Social and economic development and the fertility transitions in Mainland China and Taiwan. *Population and Development Review, 26*(Supplement), 40–60.
Rendall, M. S., Joyner, K., Peters, H. E., Yang, F., Handcock, M. S., & Ryan, A. (2006). *A Bayesian approach to combining population and survey data for male fertility estimation*. Paper presented at the Annual Meetings of Population Association of America, Los Angeles.
Singley, S. G. & Landale, N. S. (1998). Incorporating origin and process in migration fertility frameworks: The case of Puerto Rican women. *Social Forces, 76*(4), 1437–1464.
Watkins, S. (1986). Conclusions. In A. J. Coale, S. Watkins (Eds.), *The decline of fertility in Europe*. Princeton, NJ: Princeton University Press.

Index

L. Zhang, *Male Fertility Patterns and Determinants*, The Springer Series on Demographic Methods and Population Analysis 27, DOI 10.1007/978-90-481-8939-7,

FSC
www.fsc.org
MIX
Papier | Fördert gute Waldnutzung
FSC® C083411

Kolibri 360 GmbH
Ferdinand-Jühlke-Straße 7
99095 Erfurt, Deutschland
produktsicherheit@kolibri360.de